Max van Damme

Recognising Obsessive-Compulsive Disorder

A guide to self-diagnosis and understanding the symptoms

bup

Max van Damme

Recognising Obsessive-Compulsive Disorder

A guide to self-diagnosis and understanding the symptoms

ISBN: 978-3-68904-715-3
Order number: 1550 (Paperback)
Also available as an eBook

Bremen University Press, 2024.
The manuscript may not be used in whole or in part without the prior written consent of the publisher.

First edition
August 2024
bup@bremenuniversitypress.com
www.bremenuniversitypress.com

Max van Damme

Recognising Obsessive-Compulsive Disorder

A guide to self-diagnosis and understanding the symptoms

Overview

1 INTRODUCTION	5
2. BASICS OF OBSESSIVE-COMPULSIVE DISORDERS	10
3. SYMPTOMS OF OBSESSIVE-COMPULSIVE DISORDER	22
4. SELF-DIAGNOSIS: A GUIDE	36
5 DIFFERENTIATION FROM OTHER MENTAL DISORDERS	50
6 THERAPY AND TREATMENT OF OBSESSIVE-COMPULSIVE DISORDERS	71
7 PREVENTION AND EDUCATION	93
8 CONCLUSION AND OUTLOOK	109
9 FURTHER READING	115

Table of contents

1 INTRODUCTION   5

1.1 BACKGROUND AND RELEVANCE OF THE TOPIC   5
1.2 AIM AND STRUCTURE OF THE BOOK   6
1.3 METHODOLOGY AND APPROACH   8

2. BASICS OF OBSESSIVE-COMPULSIVE DISORDERS   10

2.1 DEFINITION AND CLASSIFICATION OF OBSESSIVE-COMPULSIVE DISORDER   10
2.2 HISTORICAL DEVELOPMENT AND THEORETICAL APPROACHES   12
2.3 EPIDEMIOLOGY: PREVALENCE AND RISK FACTORS   14
2.4 NEUROBIOLOGICAL AND GENETIC FOUNDATIONS   16
2.5 PSYCHOLOGICAL EXPLANATORY MODELS   19

3. SYMPTOMS OF OBSESSIVE-COMPULSIVE DISORDER   22

3.1 OBSESSIVE THOUGHTS: CHARACTERISTICS AND TYPES   22
3.2 COMPULSIVE BEHAVIOUR: FORMS AND FUNCTION   24
3.3 COGNITIVE AND EMOTIONAL SIDE EFFECTS   27
3.4 BEHAVIOUR AND EFFECTS IN EVERYDAY LIFE   30
3.5 CASE STUDIES TO ILLUSTRATE THE SYMPTOMS   32
CASE STUDY 1: ANNA, THE PERFECTIONIST   33
CASE STUDY 2: MARK, THE CLEANLINESS ADDICT   33
CASE STUDY 3: LENA, THE NEAT FREAK   34
CASE STUDY 4: THOMAS THE DOUBTER   34

4. SELF-DIAGNOSIS: A GUIDE   36

4.1 WHY SELF-DIAGNOSIS? OPPORTUNITIES AND RISKS   36
OPPORTUNITIES FOR SELF-DIAGNOSIS: 36
RISKS OF SELF-DIAGNOSIS: 37

4.2 SELF-OBSERVATION: HOW DO I RECOGNISE OBSESSIVE-COMPULSIVE SYMPTOMS? … **38**
STEPS TOWARDS SELF-OBSERVATION: … 38
4.3 VALIDATED SELF-TESTS AND QUESTIONNAIRES … **40**
EXAMPLES OF SELF-TESTS AND QUESTIONNAIRES: … 40
APPLICATION AND INTERPRETATION OF THE RESULTS: … 42
LIMITS AND CHALLENGES: … 42
4.4 LIMITS OF SELF-DIAGNOSIS: WHEN PROFESSIONAL HELP IS NECESSARY … **43**
SIGNS OF WHEN PROFESSIONAL HELP IS NEEDED: … 43
ADVANTAGES OF PROFESSIONAL DIAGNOSIS: … 44
4.5 PITFALLS AND MISINTERPRETATIONS IN SELF-DIAGNOSIS … **46**
TYPICAL PITFALLS IN SELF-DIAGNOSIS: … 46
STRATEGIES FOR AVOIDING MISINTERPRETATIONS: … 48

5 DIFFERENTIATION FROM OTHER MENTAL DISORDERS … 50

5.1 OBSESSIVE-COMPULSIVE DISORDER VS. ATTENTION-DEFICIT/HYPERACTIVITY DISORDER (ADHD) … **50**
SYMPTOM OVERLAPS: … 50
DIFFERENCES IN CAUSE AND COURSE: … 51
DIFFERENTIATION IN THE DIAGNOSTIC PROCESS: … 52
5.2 OBSESSIVE-COMPULSIVE DISORDER VS. AUTISM SPECTRUM DISORDER … **53**
TYPICAL BEHAVIOURS AND THEIR DIFFERENCES: … 53
COMMON AND DIVERGENT COGNITIVE PATTERNS: … 54
DIFFERENTIAL DIAGNOSIS: WHEN IS OBSESSIVE-COMPULSIVE DISORDER PRESENT? … 55
RESPONSE TO TREATMENT … 56
5.3 OBSESSIVE-COMPULSIVE DISORDER VS. DEPRESSION … **57**
AFFECTIVE SYMPTOMS IN COMPARISON: … 57
INTERACTIONS AND COMORBIDITIES: … 58
DIAGNOSTIC CHALLENGES AND SOLUTIONS: … 59
5.4 OBSESSIVE-COMPULSIVE DISORDER VS. BIPOLAR DISORDER … **60**
MANIC AND DEPRESSIVE PHASES: DIFFERENTIATION FROM OBSESSIVE-COMPULSIVE SYMPTOMS: … 60
COMORBID MANIFESTATIONS: … 61
DIAGNOSTIC DIFFERENTIATION AND THERAPEUTIC APPROACHES: … 62
5.5 OBSESSIVE-COMPULSIVE DISORDERS VS. ANXIETY DISORDERS … **63**
FEAR AS A COMMON DENOMINATOR? … 64
SPECIFIC DIFFERENCES IN SYMPTOMS: … 64

DIAGNOSTIC CRITERIA AND DIFFERENTIATION:	65
5.6 OBSESSIVE-COMPULSIVE DISORDERS VS. SLEEP DISORDERS	**67**
RELATIONSHIP BETWEEN SLEEP AND OBSESSIVE-COMPULSIVE SYMPTOMS:	67
SLEEP PROBLEMS AS A CONSEQUENCE OR SYMPTOM?	68
DIFFERENTIAL DIAGNOSIS AND TREATMENT APPROACHES:	69

6 THERAPY AND TREATMENT OF OBSESSIVE-COMPULSIVE DISORDERS 71

6.1 PSYCHOTHERAPY: APPROACHES AND TECHNIQUES	**71**
COGNITIVE BEHAVIOURAL THERAPY (CBT):	71
PSYCHOEDUCATION:	72
DEPTH PSYCHOLOGY-BASED THERAPY:	73
ACCEPTANCE AND COMMITMENT THERAPY (ACT):	74
6.2 DRUG TREATMENT OPTIONS	**75**
SELECTIVE SEROTONIN REUPTAKE INHIBITORS (SSRIS):	75
TRICYCLIC ANTIDEPRESSANTS (TCAS):	76
ANTIPSYCHOTICS:	77
BENZODIAZEPINES:	78
INDIVIDUAL CUSTOMISATION OF MEDICATION:	78
LONG-TERM PERSPECTIVE:	79
6.3 MULTIMODAL APPROACHES: COMBINATIONS OF FORMS OF THERAPY	**80**
COMBINATION OF PSYCHOTHERAPY AND DRUG TREATMENT:	80
INTEGRATION OF ALTERNATIVE AND COMPLEMENTARY METHODS:	81
COORDINATION OF MULTIDISCIPLINARY TEAMS:	82
LONG-TERM COPING STRATEGIES:	83
6.4 SELF-HELP AND ALTERNATIVE TREATMENT METHODS	**83**
SELF-HELP GROUPS:	84
MINDFULNESS AND MEDITATION:	84
NUTRITION AND FOOD SUPPLEMENTS:	85
PHYSICAL EXERCISE:	86
CREATIVE THERAPIES:	86
ALTERNATIVE HEALING METHODS:	87
LONG-TERM USE AND RELAPSE PREVENTION:	87
6.5 FORECAST AND LONG-TERM MANAGEMENT	**88**
LONG-TERM FORECAST:	89
RELAPSE PREVENTION:	89
STRATEGIES FOR LONG-TERM COPING:	90
MAINTAINING QUALITY OF LIFE:	91

7 PREVENTION AND EDUCATION   93

7.1 Early detection and intervention   **93**
Importance of early detection: 93
Strategies for early intervention: 94
Obstacles to early detection: 95
Measures to promote early detection: 95
7.2 Prevention programmes and educational work   **96**
Objectives of the prevention programmes: 96
Types of prevention programmes: 97
Educational work: 98
Challenges in prevention work: 99
Success criteria for prevention programmes: 99
7.3 Stigmatisation and social perception   **100**
Nature and causes of stigmatisation: 101
Effects of stigmatisation: 102
Measures to reduce stigmatisation: 102
Success criteria for anti-stigma measures: 103
7.4 Importance of social support   **104**
Forms of social support: 104
Influence of social support on treatment success: 105
Challenges in providing social support: 106
Strategies for effective social support: 107

8 CONCLUSION AND OUTLOOK   109

8.1 Summary of the key findings   **109**
8.2 Future research directions and open questions   **110**
8.3 Concluding remarks   **112**

9 FURTHER READING   115

1. introduction

1.1 Background and relevance of the topic

Obsessive-compulsive disorder (OCD) is one of the most complex and distressing mental disorders that can affect people. These disorders are characterised by the presence of obsessions and/or compulsions that severely interfere with the daily lives of those affected. Obsessive thoughts are involuntary, recurring thoughts, images or impulses that are perceived as intrusive and distressing. These thoughts generate a considerable amount of anxiety or discomfort, which leads to those affected trying to neutralise these thoughts through compulsive actions. Compulsions are repetitive, ritualised behaviours that are directly related to the obsessive thoughts and aim to reduce the discomfort caused by these thoughts.

The relevance of the topic of obsessive-compulsive disorder lies not only in the high prevalence of the disorder, which affects around 2-3% of the population worldwide, but also in the profound impairment that this disorder represents for those affected. OCD can lead to considerable social, professional and personal restrictions and is often associated with a significant deterioration in quality of life. Despite the frequency and severity of the disorder, it is often not recognised in time or misdiagnosed, partly due to the stigma attached to mental illness in general and OCD in particular.

Understanding and recognising obsessive-compulsive disorder is therefore crucial in order to be able to help sufferers at an early stage. A deeper knowledge of the symptoms, the neurobiological and psychological basis and the effective treatment methods can help to improve the quality of life of those affected and increase social acceptance of this disorder.

1.2 Aim and structure of the book

The aim of this work is to provide a comprehensive and detailed account of OCD, covering both theoretical knowledge and practical approaches to recognition, self-diagnosis and treatment. This work is aimed at a wide audience, including sufferers, family members, healthcare professionals and anyone with an interest in the subject. The aim is to provide a sound understanding of OCD, taking into account both the biological and psychological aspects of the disorder, while offering concrete guidance for self-diagnosis and differentiation from similar mental disorders.

The work is divided into several thematic chapters that gradually deepen the understanding of OCD:

- Introduction: An introduction to the topic that explains the relevance and objectives of the work.
- Basics of obsessive-compulsive disorder: This chapter deals with the definition, classification, historical development, prevalence, risk factors

and the neurobiological and psychological basis of obsessive-compulsive disorder.
- Symptoms of obsessive-compulsive disorder: A detailed description of the different types of obsessive thoughts and compulsive behaviours, including their cognitive and emotional accompaniments and their impact on daily life.
- Self-diagnosis: a guide: This chapter offers practical guidance on self-monitoring, presents validated self-tests, and discusses the limitations and risks of self-diagnosis.
- Differentiation from other mental disorders: A detailed differentiation of OCD from other mental disorders such as ADHD, autism spectrum disorder, depression and anxiety disorders.
- Therapy and treatment: A comprehensive presentation of psychotherapeutic and medicinal treatment options, including alternative and complementary approaches.
- Prevention and education: This chapter examines the importance of prevention, early detection and education as well as the role of social support.
- Conclusion and outlook: A summary of the key findings of the work, followed by an outlook on future research directions and open questions.

This structure is intended to provide the reader with an in-depth understanding of the complex subject matter, encompassing both theoretical knowledge and practical applications.

1.3 Methodology and approach

The methodology of this work is based on a comprehensive and systematic literature review, supplemented by the analysis of case studies and the evaluation of self-diagnostic instruments. The multidisciplinary approach includes the integration of findings from various fields of science, including psychology, psychiatry, neuroscience and sociology. The author himself has many years of experience in psychiatry.

- Literature research: The research included scientific articles, clinical studies, textbooks and testimonials from those affected. The selected sources came from renowned databases and journals and were chosen on the basis of specific search criteria to ensure a high level of relevance and topicality. The focus was on identifying key topics such as the aetiology, symptoms, diagnosis and treatment of OCD.
- Analysis of case studies: In order to link the theoretical findings with practical experience, several case studies were analysed. These case studies offer detailed insights into the individual experiences of those affected, the variety of symptoms and the challenges of dealing with the

disorder. They illustrate how OCD occurs in different contexts and which coping strategies can be used successfully.
- Evaluation of self-diagnostic instruments: The paper contains a critical evaluation of common self-diagnostic instruments such as the Yale-Brown Obsessive Compulsive Scale (Y-BOCS) and the Obsessive Compulsive Inventory (OCI). These instruments were analysed with regard to their validity, reliability and applicability in clinical and non-clinical settings. Analysing these instruments should help those affected to systematically record their symptoms and make an informed decision about how to proceed.
- Critical evaluation: The work includes a critical examination of the existing diagnostic and therapeutic approaches in order to highlight their strengths and weaknesses. This includes a discussion of the limitations of self-diagnosis, the challenges of differential diagnosis and the effectiveness of the various treatment methods.

This methodological approach ensures a comprehensive and well-founded investigation of obsessive-compulsive disorders that is both scientifically sound and practice-orientated.

2. basics of obsessive-compulsive disorders

2.1 Definition and classification of obsessive-compulsive disorder

Obsessive-compulsive disorder (OCD) is a class of mental disorders characterised by the presence of obsessive thoughts and/or compulsive actions. Obsessive thoughts are recurrent, intrusive thoughts, images or impulses that cause significant discomfort and are often recognised as irrational or inappropriate. Compulsions are ritualised behaviours or mental acts performed to reduce the anxiety or discomfort caused by the obsessive thoughts. These actions are not realistically related to what they claim to prevent, or they are clearly exaggerated.

Obsessive-compulsive disorders are classified in common diagnostic systems such as the Diagnostic and Statistical Manual of Mental Disorders, Fifth Edition (DSM-5), and the International Classification of Diseases, Tenth Revision (ICD-10). In the DSM-5, OCD is classified under "obsessive-compulsive and related disorders", along with other disorders such as body dysmorphic disorder and compulsive hoarding. This classification emphasises the similarities between these disorders, particularly in relation to obsessive thoughts and repetitive behaviours.

Within OCD there are different subtypes based on the predominant symptoms:

- Compulsive contamination and cleaning: This form of OCD is characterised by intense fears of contamination and the need to constantly clean oneself or one's surroundings. Those affected can spend hours washing their hands, disinfecting surfaces or performing cleaning rituals to rid themselves of the perceived danger.
- Compulsion for symmetry and order: This subtype focuses on the need for symmetry, order and precision. Those affected spend a lot of time placing objects in a certain order or carrying out actions in a certain sequence in order to avoid discomfort.
- Compulsive checking: People with this subtype have an incessant need to check things over and over again to make sure no mistakes have been made. Typical checking behaviours include repeatedly checking locks, appliances or light switches to make sure everything is secure.
- Compulsive thoughts or beliefs: This subtype is characterised by intrusive, often aggressive or inappropriate thoughts that cause anxiety. Although these thoughts are rarely translated into action, those affected feel guilty or anxious and develop mental rituals to neutralise these thoughts.

- Obsessive doubt: In this subtype, sufferers are constantly plagued by doubts about simple decisions or actions. They constantly question whether they have done something right and often repeat certain actions or seek constant reassurance to calm their doubts.

These subtypes illustrate the diversity of obsessive-compulsive disorders and the need for precise diagnostic clarification in order to enable customised treatment.

2.2 Historical development and theoretical approaches

The history of the understanding of OCD goes back a long way, and its development reflects the general progress in psychiatry and psychology. Early descriptions of obsessive thoughts and actions can be found in ancient religious and philosophical texts, where they were often interpreted as a sign of moral weakness or demonic possession. These early explanations led to people with OCD being stigmatised and ostracised.

The term "obsessive-compulsive disorder" was first systematically described in the 19th century by the French psychiatrist Jean-Étienne Dominique Esquirol. Esquirol distinguished obsessive-compulsive behaviour from other forms of madness and recognised it as a separate mental disorder. He described the symptoms as "rituals" aimed at counteracting irrational fears, thereby laying the foundation for the modern understanding of obsessive-compulsive disorder.

Sigmund Freud, the founder of psychoanalysis, made a significant contribution to the development of the theory of obsessive-compulsive disorder. Freud regarded obsessive-compulsive disorders as a form of "obsessive-compulsive neurosis" and saw them as an expression of unconscious conflicts. He postulated that obsessive thoughts and actions were symbolic expressions of repressed desires or fears rooted in early childhood. Freud's work shaped the psychoanalytical understanding of OCD for several decades, although his theories are less dominant in clinical practice today.

In the 20th century, cognitive and behavioural models were developed to explain OCD. These models, led by researchers such as Paul Salkovskis and Stanley Rachman, focused on the role of thoughts and learned behaviour in the development and maintenance of the disorder. The cognitive model postulates that OCD is caused by misinterpretations of normal thoughts that are perceived as threatening. These misinterpretations lead to increased anxiety, which is alleviated by compulsive behaviour, but this reinforces the vicious cycle of thoughts and actions.

Behavioural models complement this perspective by emphasising the role of operant conditioning. Compulsive behaviours are understood as learned behaviours that are maintained through negative reinforcement: Performing a compulsive action leads to a short-term reduction in anxiety, which stabilises and reinforces the behaviour in the long term. These models formed the basis for the development of cognitive behavioural therapy (CBT), which is now considered one of the most effective forms of treatment for OCD.

These historical and theoretical developments show how the understanding of OCD has evolved over the centuries and how different theories have contributed to today's clinical practice.

2.3 Epidemiology: prevalence and risk factors

Obsessive-compulsive disorder is a globally prevalent mental illness that can affect both adults and children. Epidemiological studies show that around 2-3% of the population will develop OCD in their lifetime. This prevalence is relatively constant across different cultures and geographical regions, suggesting universal biological and psychological mechanisms.

The disease often manifests in childhood or early adulthood, with the onset of symptoms usually occurring between the ages of 10 and 24. Men tend to develop symptoms earlier in life, while women are more commonly affected in adolescence or early adulthood. OCD is often chronic and can have a significant impact on quality of life without appropriate treatment.

Several risk factors are associated with the development of OCD:

- Genetic factors: Obsessive-compulsive disorders have a strong genetic component. First-degree relatives of sufferers have a five to ten times higher risk of also developing OCD. Twin studies show that the heritability of OCD is around 45-65%. Genetic studies have identified specific genes that are associated with an increased risk of OCD, including genes responsible for the regulation of neurotransmitters such as serotonin and glutamate.
- Environmental factors: Traumatic life events, such as abuse, neglect or the loss of a loved one, can increase the risk of developing OCD. These events can lead to a dysregulation of stress hormones and neurobiological mechanisms that favour the development of OCD.
- Neurobiological abnormalities: Studies have shown that certain brain regions, in particular the fronto-striatal circuit, are overactive in people with OCD. These regions are responsible for impulse control, action planning and error processing. Dysregulation of the serotonergic system, which is responsible for the regulation of mood and anxiety, has also been demonstrated in OCD.
- Personality traits: Certain personality traits, such as perfectionism, an increased assumption of responsibility and a tendency towards excessive self-control, are often found in people with OCD. These characteristics can increase susceptibility

to obsessive thoughts and actions and favour the maintenance of the disorder.

Obsessive-compulsive disorders often occur co-morbidly with other mental disorders, such as depression, anxiety disorders, eating disorders or substance abuse disorders. These comorbidities can complicate the course and treatment of OCD and require a comprehensive, interdisciplinary treatment strategy.

2.4 Neurobiological and genetic foundations

The neurobiological basis of OCD is the subject of intensive research, as a better understanding of these mechanisms could open up new possibilities for treatment and prevention. One of the central hypotheses in this area concerns the dysfunction of the fronto-striatal circuit, which plays a key role in impulse control, action planning and error processing.

- Fronto-striatal circuit: This neural circuit comprises several brain regions, including the orbitofrontal cortex (OFC), the anterior cingulate cortex (ACC) and the caudate nucleus. People with OCD have been found to have excessive activity in these regions, leading to difficulties in suppressing unwanted thoughts and flexibility of behavioural patterns. This overactivity could explain why

obsessive thoughts are so persistent and difficult to ignore.
- Serotonergic system: Serotonin is a neurotransmitter that plays an important role in regulating mood, anxiety and impulse control. Studies have shown that there is a dysregulation of the serotonergic system in people with obsessive-compulsive disorder. This dysregulation could contribute to the pronounced anxiety symptoms and compulsive behaviour. The efficacy of SSRIs (selective serotonin reuptake inhibitors) in the treatment of OCD supports the hypothesis that the serotonergic system plays a central role in the pathophysiology of the disorder.
- Glutamatergic system: Recent research suggests that the glutamatergic system, which is responsible for the transmission of excitation in the brain, may also play a role in OCD. Studies have shown that genetic variants that influence the function of glutamate transport are associated with an increased risk of obsessive-compulsive disorder. Dysregulation of glutamate transport could lead to overexcitation of certain brain regions responsible for controlling thoughts and behaviour.
- Genetic predisposition: OCD is strongly influenced by genetics, and several genes have been identified that are associated with an increased risk of developing the disorder.

These include genes that are important for the function of neurotransmitters such as serotonin, glutamate and dopamine. These genetic predispositions could cause certain areas of the brain to be hypersensitive to stimuli and the brain to have difficulty suppressing inappropriate thoughts or behaviours.

- Neuroimaging studies: Imaging techniques such as functional magnetic resonance imaging (fMRI) and positron emission tomography (PET) have provided important insights into brain activity in OCD. These studies show that sufferers have increased activity in the above-mentioned brain regions, particularly in situations that trigger obsessive thoughts. These findings support the hypothesis that OCD is associated with dysfunction in the circuits responsible for impulse control and the response to fear.

Research into the neurobiological and genetic basis of OCD helps to better understand the complexity of the disorder and identify potential targets for new therapeutic approaches. A deeper understanding of these mechanisms could in future lead to the development of personalised treatment strategies that are tailored to the individual neurobiological profiles of those affected.

2.5 Psychological explanatory models

The psychological explanatory models for OCD offer valuable insights into the cognitive and emotional processes that contribute to the development and maintenance of the disorder. These models help to understand the mechanisms by which normal thoughts become distressing obsessive thoughts and how ritualised behaviours emerge and are reinforced.

- Cognitive model: The cognitive model of OCD, developed by researchers such as Paul Salkovskis, emphasises the role of misinterpretations and irrational beliefs in the development of obsessive thoughts. This model postulates that obsessive thoughts can occur in all people, but in people with OCD these thoughts are perceived as particularly threatening or meaningful. These misinterpretations lead to a sense of excessive responsibility that forces the person to perform ritualised actions to prevent the feared event. For example, a person who believes that the mere thought of harming someone could actually cause harm may develop obsessive control rituals to avoid this danger.
- Behavioural model: The behavioural model, which is based on classical and operant conditioning, explains OCD as a learned response to fear. In this model, the compulsive action is seen as a reaction to a fear-inducing stimulus that is maintained through negative reinforcement.

Each time a compulsive action is performed, it reduces anxiety in the short term, which increases the likelihood that the action will be repeated in the future. This reinforcement leads to the compulsive actions becoming more frequent and intense until they dominate a large part of the sufferer's life.

- Metacognitive model: This model extends the cognitive model by focussing on the role of metacognition, i.e. thoughts about thoughts. The metacognitive model assumes that people with OCD not only perceive their obsessive thoughts as threatening, but also believe that they need to control their thoughts. This belief leads to a vicious cycle in which attempts to suppress obsessive thoughts actually lead to an increase in these thoughts. These increased obsessive thoughts in turn reinforce the feeling of losing control, forcing sufferers to intensify their efforts to control their thoughts.

- Emotional processing theories: These theories emphasise the role of emotional processing in OCD. They postulate that obsessive thoughts are often associated with intense negative emotions such as fear, guilt or disgust, which sufferers are unable to fully process. In order to cope with these negative emotions, they develop compulsive behaviours that provide short-term relief but hinder emotional processing in the long term. This theory suggests that OCD has not only

a cognitive but also an emotional component that must be taken into account in treatment.
- Psychoanalytic theories: Although less prominent today, psychoanalytic theories continue to offer a perspective on OCD that focuses on unconscious conflicts and early childhood. In these theories, obsessive thoughts and actions are understood as expressions of repressed desires or fears that have their origins in early childhood experiences. These conflicts are symbolically expressed through compulsive rituals, which serve both as defence mechanisms against the threatening desires and as an attempt to maintain control over these desires.

These psychological explanatory models are not just theoretical constructs, but have practical implications for the treatment of OCD. They form the basis for various therapeutic approaches, particularly cognitive behavioural therapy, which focuses on changing the cognitive and behavioural patterns that maintain OCD. A deeper understanding of these models can help to develop customised treatment plans that are tailored to the specific needs and thought patterns of those affected.

3. symptoms of obsessive-compulsive disorder

3.1 Obsessive thoughts: characteristics and types

Obsessive thoughts are a central feature of obsessive-compulsive disorders and can occur in various forms. They are typically unwanted, intrusive and cause considerable discomfort to those affected. Although the content of the obsessive thoughts can vary, they all have in common that they are perceived as irrational or exaggerated, but this does not prevent them from being very distressing for the person affected.

- Contamination thoughts: This type of obsessive thoughts refers to the fear of contamination or contamination by dirt, germs, chemicals or other potentially dangerous substances. People affected by these thoughts fear that they or others could become ill if they come into contact with certain substances or objects. These thoughts often lead to compulsive hand washing, cleaning rituals or avoidance of certain places and situations that are considered contaminated.
- Aggressive obsessive thoughts: This form of obsessive thoughts involves intrusive thoughts of hurting someone or harming oneself. These thoughts are particularly frightening as they often contradict the moral beliefs and values of

those affected. Despite the intense fear that these thoughts evoke, in most cases there is no actual danger of the person concerned acting on their thoughts. Nevertheless, these thoughts can cause sufferers to withdraw from other people to ensure that they do not harm anyone.

- Obsessive sexual thoughts: These thoughts are unwanted and intrusive sexual fantasies or images that are perceived as inappropriate or repulsive. For example, sufferers may have recurring thoughts of sexual acts that are considered morally reprehensible or inappropriate. These thoughts often lead to intense feelings of guilt and shame and can cause sufferers to completely repress or overly control their sexuality.
- Religious or blasphemous obsessive thoughts: These thoughts concern the fear of violating religious commandments or having blasphemous thoughts. People who suffer from these thoughts may fear that they are committing sins or betraying their faith through their thoughts. These thoughts often lead to excessive praying, confession or other religious rituals to atone for the perceived guilt.
- Symmetry and order compulsion thoughts: These thoughts relate to the need for symmetry, order and perfection. Affected people may think incessantly about how to align objects, perform steps in a certain order or ensure that everything is "perfect". These thoughts can become so

intense that they significantly disrupt daily life, as sufferers spend a lot of time trying to fulfil these requirements.
- Obsessive doubts: This type of obsessive thoughts involves constant doubt and uncertainty about everyday actions. People with obsessive doubts may wonder whether they have really locked a door, switched off the cooker or done something wrong. These doubts lead to repeated checking and the need to constantly reassure themselves that everything is OK.

These different types of obsessive thoughts show how varied and stressful the thoughts of people with OCD can be. Despite their differences, what all these thoughts have in common is that they are perceived by those affected as disturbing, inappropriate and difficult to control, which can lead to considerable emotional and social problems.

3.2 Compulsive behaviour: Forms and function

Compulsions are the repeated behaviours or mental acts that are performed in response to obsessive thoughts. The main function of these acts is to reduce the anxiety caused by the obsessive thoughts or to prevent a feared misfortune. Although compulsive behaviours can bring short-term relief, in the long term they reinforce the obsessive thoughts and make the disorder worse.

- Cleaning rituals: Cleaning compulsions are a common form of compulsive behaviour, especially in people with contamination anxiety. These rituals can include hours of hand washing, showering or cleaning objects. Those affected often wash in a certain order or according to certain rules to ensure that they are "clean". These rituals can become so time-consuming that they significantly interfere with daily life, and they often lead to physical damage such as skin irritations or infections.

- Control rituals: People with control compulsions repeatedly check whether they have carried out everyday tasks correctly, such as locking doors, switching off electrical appliances or writing emails. These actions are usually repeated several times, as those affected have the feeling that they have overlooked something or that a mistake could have fatal consequences. These control rituals can lead to those affected being late for work, avoiding social activities or being unable to complete their tasks efficiently.
- Counting rituals: Counting compulsions involve the need to do or count certain things a certain number of times. For example, sufferers may count steps before entering a room or count letters in a sentence to ensure they don't reach an 'unlucky' number. These rituals are often

performed in a set order and are difficult to interrupt without causing significant anxiety.
- Ordering and symmetry: Compulsive behaviours that focus on order and symmetry involve arranging objects according to certain rules so that they are perfectly aligned or symmetrical. Affected people spend a lot of time making sure that all objects in their environment are arranged "correctly" and can become very stressed if something is not perfect. These actions can extend to all aspects of life, from the organisation of the workplace to the arrangement of food in the fridge.
- Mental rituals: In addition to physical compulsions, there are also mental rituals in which those affected try to neutralise their obsessive thoughts through certain mental processes. These include, for example, repeating certain words or sentences, mentally "going through" actions to ensure that they have been performed correctly, or visualising positive images to "erase" negative thoughts. These mental rituals are often less obvious, but can be just as time-consuming and stressful as physical compulsions.
- Avoidance: Another form of compulsive behaviour is the avoidance of situations that could trigger obsessive thoughts. People with obsessive-compulsive disorder often develop complex strategies to avoid triggers, which can lead to a considerable restriction of their lives. This

avoidance can go so far that sufferers limit their social contacts, neglect their work or avoid public places.

Compulsive behaviours are often distressing for sufferers as they feel they have no control over their actions and that these actions are necessary to relieve their anxiety. These rituals are not only time-consuming, but can also lead to considerable physical and psychological stress, which emphasises the need for effective treatment.

3.3 Cognitive and emotional side effects

OCD is characterised not only by obsessive thoughts and actions, but also by a range of cognitive distortions and emotional reactions that maintain and exacerbate the disorder. These concomitants play a central role in the experience of people with OCD and influence how they perceive and respond to their thoughts, feelings and actions.

- Exaggerated responsibility: One of the most common cognitive distortions in OCD is the belief that one is overly responsible for the well-being of others. People with OCD tend to believe that they could cause harm through their thoughts or actions and that it is their duty to prevent this from happening. This exaggerated responsibility leads them to perform ritualised

actions to ensure that they do not do anything 'wrong', causing considerable stress and discomfort.
- Perfectionism: Many people with OCD have a pronounced perfectionism that drives them to complete all tasks flawlessly. This perfectionism can extend to all areas of life, from work and personal life to everyday tasks. The constant striving for perfection often leads to self-doubt and the feeling that one is never doing enough, which can lead to an increase in compulsive behaviour.
- Magical thinking: Magical thinking is the irrational belief that thoughts or actions can supernaturally influence real events. People with OCD may believe that certain thoughts or rituals are necessary to prevent disasters. For example, they may think that counting a certain number of steps could prevent something bad from happening. This form of thinking reinforces the compulsive behaviour and makes it difficult to overcome the disorder.
- Anxiety and panic: Anxiety is a central emotional symptom of obsessive-compulsive disorder. Obsessive thoughts often trigger intense anxiety or even panic, as they are perceived as a threat. This fear leads to an urgent need to perform compulsive actions in order to neutralise the feared danger. The constant anxiety and stress associated with OCD can lead to a state of chronic tension and exhaustion.

- Guilt and shame: Many people with OCD struggle with strong feelings of guilt and shame. They often feel guilty for their obsessive thoughts, especially if they are aggressive, sexual or blasphemous. These thoughts are at odds with the sufferer's moral convictions, which leads to intense feelings of shame and self-condemnation. These emotions can further intensify the obsessive thoughts and actions, as sufferers try to "atone" for their guilt through even more rigorous rituals.
- Constant doubt and uncertainty: Obsessive-compulsive disorder is often accompanied by a constant feeling of uncertainty and doubt. Those affected have difficulty making decisions or feeling sure that they have done something right. This insecurity leads to repeated checking and the need to constantly seek reassurance, which reinforces the compulsive behaviour.

These cognitive and emotional side effects make it clear that OCD goes far beyond simple behaviours and is deeply rooted in the thought patterns and emotional reactions of those affected. Successful treatment must therefore address not only the compulsive behaviours, but also the underlying cognitive distortions and emotional difficulties that perpetuate the disorder.

3.4 Behaviour and effects in everyday life

Obsessive-compulsive disorders have a profound impact on the daily lives of those affected and can lead to considerable restrictions in almost all areas of life. Obsessive thoughts and actions often take up so much time and energy that normal everyday activities are neglected. The effects on behaviour and quality of life are considerable and range from social and professional problems to physical and mental health problems.

- Work and school performance: People with OCD often find it difficult to fulfil their tasks at school or at work. Obsessive behaviours such as constant checking, cleaning or tidying can take up so much time that those affected are unable to complete their work on time. Obsessive thoughts can also impair concentration and decision-making, leading to errors and reduced productivity. This in turn can lead to conflicts with colleagues, superiors or teachers and, in extreme cases, even to job loss or academic failure.
- Social isolation: The fear that other people will notice their obsessive-compulsive symptoms or that they will find themselves in situations that trigger their compulsive behaviour often leads those affected to withdraw socially. They may avoid social contact, parties or other events for fear that they will not be able to hide their compulsive behaviour or that their rituals will be interrupted by others. This withdrawal leads to

loneliness and can increase the feeling of isolation, which in turn can exacerbate the obsessive-compulsive symptoms.
- Interpersonal relationships: OCD can cause considerable tension in interpersonal relationships. Partners, family members and friends may perceive the rituals and behaviours of those affected as irrational or distressing, which can lead to conflict. In many cases, family members try to support or facilitate the compulsive behaviour of those affected in order to avoid conflict, but this often leads to the disorder being perpetuated. In other cases, the lack of understanding or frustration of relatives can lead to a deterioration in relationships and even to their breakdown.
- Physical health: The physical effects of OCD can also be significant. Excessive hand washing or cleaning can lead to skin irritation, eczema or infection. Compulsive behaviours such as counting or repeating movements can lead to physical exhaustion or injury. In addition, the constant anxiety and chronic stress associated with OCD can lead to a variety of stress-related physical ailments, including headaches, gastrointestinal problems and sleep disorders.
- Financial problems: In some cases, OCD can lead to financial difficulties. For example, those suffering from a compulsion to clean may buy excessive amounts of cleaning products or use expensive cleaning services. Others may find it

difficult to hold down a regular job due to their compulsive behaviours, leading to loss of income and financial problems.
- Impact on self-image: People with OCD often develop a negative self-image characterised by guilt, shame and feelings of inadequacy. They may feel worthless or unable to control their obsessive thoughts and actions, which can lead to reduced self-esteem and depression. These negative feelings can further exacerbate the disorder and make it difficult for sufferers to seek help.

The effects of OCD on daily life are varied and far-reaching. They affect not only the sufferers themselves, but also their surroundings and social environment. Effective treatment must therefore take all these aspects into account in order to improve the quality of life of those affected and help them to lead a fulfilling and productive life.

3.5 Case studies to illustrate the symptoms

To illustrate the variety and intensity of the symptoms of OCD, this section presents case studies that illustrate the different forms of the disorder and their impact on the lives of those affected.

Case study 1: Anna, the perfectionist

Anna is a 32-year-old teacher who has suffered from obsessive-compulsive disorder since her youth. Her main symptoms are obsessive doubt and perfectionism. Anna often spends hours preparing teaching materials and making sure they are error-free. Despite her efforts, she constantly feels that something is not right and checks her work over and over again. This perfectionism not only affects her professional performance, but also leads to a lack of sleep and exhaustion, as Anna often works late into the night. Her OCD has caused her to isolate herself socially, as she has little time for friends or leisure activities. Despite the stress, Anna finds it difficult to control her symptoms as she fears that she could make a mistake that would jeopardise her career.

Case study 2: Mark, the cleanliness addict

Markus is a 28-year-old IT specialist who suffers from a severe form of contamination anxiety. His obsessive thoughts constantly revolve around the fear of becoming infected with dangerous germs. Markus spends several hours a day washing his hands, sanitising his home and cleaning his clothes. He avoids public transport, public toilets and avoids touching people for fear of contamination. These rituals have severely restricted Markus' life; he works from home and rarely leaves his flat. His OCD has also caused problems in his relationship, as his partner has difficulty coping with his extreme cleaning rituals.

Case study 3: Lena, the neat freak

Lena is a 40-year-old mother of two who suffers from a severe obsession with tidiness. Lena spends several hours a day making sure that all the objects in her house are perfectly aligned and symmetrical. She has developed specific rituals to ensure that everything is "just right" and becomes extremely anxious and irritable if anything is out of balance. Her OCD has meant that she often criticises her children when they make the house 'messy', which has caused tension in the family. Lena knows that her OCD behaviours are irrational, but she feels compelled to carry them out to relieve her anxiety.

Case study 4: Thomas the doubter

Thomas is a 35-year-old lawyer who suffers from obsessive doubts. He spends hours every day checking whether he has filled out important documents correctly, worded emails correctly and made legal decisions correctly. These constant doubts cause him to constantly revise his work and hesitate to make decisions for fear of making a mistake. Thomas' OCD has seriously affected his career as he often misses deadlines and fails to meet important deadlines. He feels constantly stressed and overwhelmed, which has led to a decline in his job performance and a loss of self-confidence.

These case studies show the many forms that OCD can take and the profound impact it has on the lives of those affected. They illustrate how obsessive thoughts and actions can dominate daily life and lead to considerable social, professional and personal restrictions. These examples also emphasise the need for individualised and comprehensive treatment that is tailored to the specific needs of those affected.

4. self-diagnosis: a guide

4.1 Why self-diagnosis? Opportunities and risks

Self-diagnosis of mental disorders, especially obsessive-compulsive disorder, is a double-edged sword. On the one hand, it can be a valuable tool for developing an awareness of one's own symptoms, but on the other hand it harbours considerable risks, especially if it is carried out without professional support.

Opportunities for self-diagnosis:

- Early detection: One of the greatest opportunities for self-diagnosis lies in the early detection of OCD. Often people are not able to recognise their symptoms immediately or they only seek help late, when the symptoms are already severe. Self-diagnosis can alert sufferers to possible signs at an early stage, which can lead to faster intervention.
- Self-awareness and empowerment: By dealing with their own symptoms, sufferers can develop a better understanding of their own thoughts and behaviour patterns. This can lead to them feeling more responsible for their own health and actively seeking solutions.
- First steps to help: Self-diagnosis can be the first step to seeking professional help. Many people

are reluctant to see a therapist or doctor because they don't take their symptoms seriously enough or believe they don't need help. A self-diagnosis can help them overcome their concerns and give them the courage to seek professional help.

Risks of self-diagnosis:

- Misdiagnosis: One of the biggest risks of self-diagnosis is the possibility of misdiagnosis. OCD shares many symptoms with other mental disorders, such as anxiety disorders, depression or obsessive-compulsive disorder. Without the necessary expertise, sufferers may misinterpret their symptoms, which can lead to inappropriate or delayed treatment.
- Overdiagnosis: On the other hand, there is a risk that those affected may believe that they have a more serious disorder than is actually the case due to a self-diagnosis. This can lead to unnecessary anxiety and stress and cause them to overburden themselves or undergo inappropriate treatment methods.
- Avoiding professional help: Another risk is that sufferers believe they can manage their symptoms alone without recognising the need for professional help. This can lead to them not receiving appropriate treatment and their symptoms worsening.

- Self-stigmatisation: Self-diagnosis can also lead to self-stigmatisation, especially if sufferers believe that their symptoms make them weak or "abnormal". This can undermine self-esteem and increase feelings of isolation.

Overall, self-diagnosis should be seen as a potentially helpful but also dangerous tool. It is important that sufferers who self-diagnose realise that this can only be a first step and that confirmation and further treatment by a qualified professional is essential.

4.2 Self-observation: How do I recognise obsessive-compulsive symptoms?

Self-observation is an important method for recognising and better understanding obsessive-compulsive symptoms. It requires a systematic and mindful approach in which those affected learn to consciously perceive and document their thoughts, feelings and behaviour.

Steps towards self-observation:

- Identification of triggers: The first step is to identify the triggers for obsessive thoughts and actions. Triggers can be certain situations, places, people or thoughts that trigger the obsessive-compulsive symptoms. Those affected should make a note of the situations in which their

symptoms occur particularly strongly and what these situations have in common.
- Observation of frequency and intensity: It is important to observe the frequency and intensity of obsessive thoughts and actions. Those affected can keep a diary in which they record how often certain thoughts or actions occur, how strong the associated anxiety is and how long the symptoms last. These records can later serve as a valuable tool for therapy.
- Differentiating between normal thoughts and obsessive thoughts: Another important step is to differentiate between normal, everyday thoughts and obsessive thoughts. Obsessive thoughts are typically intrusive, uncontrollable and cause considerable discomfort. They often contradict the moral convictions of those affected and are perceived as irrational.
- Reflect on the impact on daily life: Sufferers should ask themselves how their obsessive thoughts and actions affect their daily lives. Do the symptoms affect their work, social relationships or leisure activities? Do they spend a lot of time carrying out their obsessive behaviours? This reflection can help to recognise the extent of the disorder and assess how much it is affecting their lives.
- Self-acceptance and patience: An important aspect of self-observation is accepting your own symptoms and developing patience with

yourself. OCD is a mental illness and it is important to remember that you are not responsible for your thoughts and actions. Self-observation should not lead to additional stress or self-judgement, but should be seen as a means of self-awareness and self-care.
- Through systematic self-observation, sufferers can develop a deeper understanding of their obsessive-compulsive symptoms and be better able to control their thoughts and behaviour. This method can also help to raise awareness of patterns and triggers that can be further analysed and worked on in therapy.

4.3 Validated self-tests and questionnaires

Validated self-tests and questionnaires are important tools for the self-assessment of OCD. They offer a structured way to assess the severity of symptoms and provide clues as to whether a professional diagnosis is necessary. These instruments have been scientifically developed and have proven to be reliable and valid in the assessment of obsessive-compulsive symptoms.

Examples of self-tests and questionnaires:

- Yale-Brown Obsessive Compulsive Scale (Y-BOCS): The Y-BOCS is one of the most commonly used questionnaires for assessing obsessive-compulsive disorder. It consists of two

parts: a symptom checklist that asks about different types of obsessive thoughts and actions, and a scale that rates the severity of symptoms. Sufferers are asked to indicate how much time they spend each day with obsessive thoughts and actions, how much distress they cause and how much they interfere with daily life. The Y-BOCS can be used both for self-assessment and in a clinical setting to determine the severity of the disorder.
- Obsessive Compulsive Inventory-Revised (OCI-R): The OCI-R is another validated questionnaire developed to assess the presence and severity of obsessive-compulsive symptoms. It includes several subscales that cover different types of obsessive thoughts and actions, such as washing, checking, organising and counting. The OCI-R is easy to administer and can be a useful adjunct to clinical assessment.
- Beck Anxiety Inventory (BAI): Although the BAI was not developed specifically for OCD, it is useful for measuring the level of anxiety associated with OCD symptoms. Since anxiety plays a central role in OCD, the BAI can help determine the severity of anxiety and assess how much it affects daily life.
- Patient Health Questionnaire (PHQ-9): The PHQ-9 is a short questionnaire that measures the severity of depression. As OCD is often associated with depression, this questionnaire can help

to identify comorbid depressive symptoms that also need to be treated.

Application and interpretation of the results:

The results of these self-tests should be seen as an indication and not as a definitive diagnosis. They provide a snapshot of symptoms and can help you to develop a better understanding of your own condition. However, it is important to emphasise that self-diagnosis using these tools is not a substitute for professional diagnosis and treatment. The results should be discussed with a qualified therapist or psychiatrist who is able to make a comprehensive assessment and develop an appropriate treatment plan.

Limits and challenges:

While validated self-tests can be valuable tools, there are also limitations and challenges to their use. For one, they can be subjective as they are based on self-reporting. This can lead to bias, especially if sufferers downplay or exaggerate their symptoms. In addition, these tests do not always capture the full complexity of OCD, especially when rare or atypical symptoms are present. Therefore, the results should always be seen in the context of a comprehensive clinical assessment.

4.4 Limits of self-diagnosis: when professional help is necessary

Self-diagnosis of OCD can be helpful in recognising the first signs and becoming aware of your own situation. However, there are clear limits beyond which professional help becomes essential. It is important to know when self-diagnosis reaches its limits and a sound diagnostic clarification by a specialist is necessary.

Signs of when professional help is needed:

- Severity of the symptoms: If the obsessive-compulsive symptoms are severe and significantly interfere with daily life, professional help should be sought urgently. Signs of severe obsessive-compulsive disorder include: Obsessive thoughts that take up most of the day, compulsive behaviours that take up several hours a day, and significant interference with social, work or school activities.
- Comorbidities: Obsessive-compulsive disorders often occur together with other mental disorders, such as depression, anxiety disorders or eating disorders. If there are signs of another mental disorder alongside the obsessive-compulsive symptoms, a professional assessment is essential. Co-morbid disorders can complicate the course of OCD and require a comprehensive treatment strategy.

- Self-harming behaviour or suicidal thoughts: If those affected develop self-harming behaviour or suicidal thoughts, immediate professional help is required. These symptoms indicate a serious mental health crisis that needs to be treated immediately.
- Inability to control compulsive behaviour: If sufferers find that they can no longer control their compulsive behaviours despite their best efforts, professional help should be sought. OCD can worsen over time and without appropriate treatment there is a risk that the symptoms will get out of control.
- Misinterpretation of symptoms: If sufferers have difficulty interpreting their symptoms correctly, or if they are unsure whether they are actually suffering from OCD, it is important to seek professional clarification. OCD can easily be confused with other mental disorders and an accurate diagnosis is crucial for choosing the right treatment.

Advantages of professional diagnosis:

A professional diagnosis offers several advantages that go beyond the possibilities of self-diagnosis. A qualified professional can:

- Carry out a comprehensive assessment: This includes not only recording the symptoms, but

also examining the patient's medical history, family history and current life situation. This holistic approach enables a more precise diagnosis and individualised treatment planning.
- Make a differential diagnosis: A professional will be able to differentiate OCD from other mental disorders that have similar symptoms, such as generalised anxiety disorder, depression or obsessive-compulsive disorder. This is crucial to ensure that treatment is tailored to the specific disorder.
- Develop a personalised treatment plan: Based on the diagnosis, a professional can create a personalised treatment plan that may include both psychotherapeutic and medication approaches. This ensures that the treatment is tailored to the individual's needs and offers the best possible chance of success.
- Offer long-term support: OCD is often chronic and requires long-term support. A professional can provide ongoing support to prevent relapses and monitor the progress of treatment.

Overall, it is important that sufferers recognise the limitations of self-diagnosis and know when it is necessary to seek professional help. Early intervention by a qualified professional can be crucial in alleviating symptoms and improving the quality of life of those affected.

4.5 Pitfalls and misinterpretations in self-diagnosis

Self-diagnosis of OCD can be associated with various pitfalls and misinterpretations that can interfere with understanding one's symptoms and the path to proper treatment. It is important to be aware of these pitfalls in order to make the most accurate self-assessment and smooth the transition to professional help.

Typical pitfalls in self-diagnosis:

- Confusion with other mental disorders: OCD shares symptoms with a number of other mental disorders, such as generalised anxiety disorder, depression, post-traumatic stress disorder (PTSD) or obsessive-compulsive disorder. It can be difficult to distinguish between these disorders, especially without in-depth expertise. For example, constant worry and excessive anxiety can occur in both OCD and generalised anxiety disorder, but the underlying mechanisms and treatment differ.
- Normalising symptoms: A common pitfall in self-diagnosis is the tendency to dismiss obsessive-compulsive symptoms as normal behaviours or idiosyncrasies. Sufferers may think that their obsessive thoughts are just "overly cautious" or that their compulsive behaviours are "harmless habits". This normalisation can lead to

symptoms going untreated and worsening over time.
- Overdiagnosis: On the other hand, there is a risk of overdiagnosis, where normal worries or behaviours are misinterpreted as OCD. For example, someone who occasionally takes great care to ensure that everything is tidy may believe that they suffer from obsessive-compulsive disorder. Such misinterpretations can cause unnecessary stress and lead sufferers to focus excessively on symptoms that may not be pathological.
- Self-stigmatisation and anxiety: Self-diagnosis can lead to self-stigmatisation, in which those affected perceive themselves as "ill" or "disturbed". This can significantly affect self-esteem and lead to an increase in symptoms. In addition, the fear of actually suffering from a mental disorder can lead sufferers to over-interpret their symptoms and develop additional anxiety.
- Overlooking comorbid disorders: When self-diagnosing, there is a risk of overlooking comorbid disorders. OCD often co-occurs with other mental disorders, such as depression, anxiety disorders or substance abuse disorders. These co-morbid conditions can exacerbate the symptoms of OCD and require specific treatment that goes beyond simply treating the OCD symptoms.

Strategies for avoiding misinterpretations:

- Education and awareness: One of the best ways to avoid misinterpretation is to educate yourself about OCD and other mental disorders. Understanding the typical symptoms, causes and treatment options can help to make a more accurate self-assessment.
- Self-reflection: It is important to critically scrutinise yourself and reflect on whether the perceived symptoms actually fit into the framework of an obsessive-compulsive disorder or whether they may have other causes. You should be aware that it is normal to worry occasionally or to repeat certain behaviours without this being pathological.
- Use of self-tests in conjunction with professional counselling: Self-tests and questionnaires can provide valuable information, but should always be used in combination with professional counselling. If the results of self-tests indicate a possible OCD, it is advisable to discuss them with a therapist or psychiatrist who can make an accurate diagnosis.
- Openness to professional help: If there are uncertainties or doubts about your own diagnosis, you should be open to seeking professional help. A qualified specialist can help to correctly interpret the symptoms and develop the right treatment strategy.

Overall, it is important to consider self-diagnosis as a potentially useful but also limited tool. Whilst it can help to create an initial awareness of possible OCD, it is not an alternative to professional diagnosis and treatment. By avoiding the aforementioned pitfalls and taking a reflective approach, sufferers can make a more accurate self-assessment and facilitate the transition to appropriate treatment.

5. differentiation from other mental disorders

5.1 Obsessive-compulsive disorder vs. attention-deficit/hyperactivity disorder (ADHD)

Obsessive-compulsive disorder (OCD) and attention-deficit/hyperactivity disorder (ADHD) are two different mental disorders, but they can overlap in certain symptoms. This overlap can make diagnosis more difficult, which is why careful differentiation is necessary.

Symptom overlaps:

- Restlessness and difficulty concentrating: Both ADHD and OCD sufferers can have difficulties concentrating and staying focussed. In ADHD, this inattention often results from a fundamental difficulty in filtering stimuli and focussing on a task, whereas in OCD it often results from constant distraction by obsessive thoughts. Those affected may be so engrossed in their thoughts and rituals that they have difficulty concentrating on other tasks.
- Impulsivity vs. compulsivity: Another common characteristic can be apparent impulsivity in behaviour. In ADHD, this manifests itself as actual impulsivity, where sufferers act without much thought, which can lead to mistakes or

inappropriate behaviour. OCD, on the other hand, is a type of "compulsive impulsivity" where sufferers feel compelled to perform certain actions to relieve anxiety or discomfort. However, these actions are less spontaneous and more characterised by rigid, ritualised patterns.

Differences in cause and course:

- Neurobiological differences: ADHD is a neurodevelopmental disorder caused by abnormalities in the function of the dopaminergic and noradrenergic systems in the brain. These abnormalities primarily affect the prefrontal cortex, which is responsible for executive functions such as planning, impulse control and attention. Obsessive-compulsive disorders, on the other hand, tend to be associated with dysfunction of the fronto-striatal circuitry and the serotonergic system, which affects impulse control and the response to anxiety.
- Course and prognosis: ADHD typically begins in childhood and can continue into adulthood, while OCD usually begins somewhat later, often in adolescence or early adulthood. The course of ADHD is often stable, while OCD can worsen over time, especially if left untreated. However, both disorders can be chronic and require long-term treatment.

Differentiation in the diagnostic process:

- Diagnostic criteria: The diagnosis of ADHD is based on the presence of symptoms in the areas of inattention, hyperactivity and impulsivity that persist over a longer period of time and occur in different areas of life (e.g. school, work, home). Obsessive-compulsive disorder, on the other hand, is diagnosed on the basis of recurring obsessive thoughts and compulsive behaviour that cause considerable anxiety and severely interfere with daily life.
- Clinical interviews and scales: Differentiating between the two disorders often requires the use of specialised diagnostic tools, such as clinical interviews and validated scales. The Conners' Adult ADHD Rating Scale (CAARS) or the ADHD Rating Scale (ADHD-RS) can be used to measure the severity of ADHD symptoms. At the same time, the Yale-Brown Obsessive Compulsive Scale (Y-BOCS) can be used to assess the severity of obsessive-compulsive disorder.
- Medical and life history: A comprehensive medical history is crucial in order to understand the development of symptoms over time. In ADHD, a family history of hyperactivity and impulsivity is often reported, while in OCD there is often a family history of anxiety disorders or depression. It is also important to note that ADHD is often associated with learning difficulties and

academic problems, while OCD has a greater impact on the emotional and social domains.

The distinction between OCD and ADHD is crucial, as the treatment approaches are different. While ADHD is often treated with stimulants such as methylphenidate or amphetamines, the treatment of OCD usually requires a combination of cognitive behavioural therapy and medication with SSRIs. An accurate diagnosis is therefore essential to ensure that sufferers receive the appropriate treatment.

5.2 Obsessive-compulsive disorder vs. autism spectrum disorder

OCD and autism spectrum disorders (ASD) share some similar characteristics, particularly in terms of repetitive behaviours and rigid thought patterns. This can make it difficult to differentiate between the two disorders, especially in people who show both obsessive-compulsive symptoms and autistic traits.

Typical behaviours and their differences:

- Repetitive behaviours: Both people with OCD and people with ASD often exhibit repetitive behaviours. However, in OCD, these behaviours are usually ritualised and performed to alleviate a specific fear or discomfort (e.g. washing hands to reduce fear of contamination). In ASD,

repetitive behaviours are often performed for self-regulation, sensory pleasure or to maintain stability and predictability in their environment (e.g. repeatedly spinning objects or arranging toys in a consistent manner).
- Stereotypies and compulsive behaviours: Stereotypies are repetitive movements or vocalisations that are common in people with ASD and have no specific purpose, except possibly to satisfy sensory needs or relieve stress. Compulsions, on the other hand, are purposeful actions aimed at neutralising a fear or preventing a feared event. For example, a child with ASD might repeatedly flap their hands, while a child with OCD might repeatedly wash their hands to "cleanse" themselves of a feared contamination.

Common and divergent cognitive patterns:

- Cognitive rigidity: Both disorders are characterised by cognitive rigidity, but the way in which this rigidity manifests itself differs. People with OCD tend to hold on to irrational beliefs or fears that they try to manage through ritualised actions. People with ASD may also have rigid thought patterns, but these are often based on the need to maintain order and predictability in their environment to avoid anxiety and confusion. This rigidity can manifest itself in a preference

for routine, resistance to change and a restricted range of interests.
- Theory of mind and social cognition: A key difference between OCD and ASD lies in social cognition. People with ASD often have difficulty understanding the thoughts, feelings and intentions of others (theory of mind), which can lead to social misunderstandings and difficulties in interpersonal relationships. In people with OCD, social cognition is usually intact, but they may withdraw socially due to their OCD symptoms or worry excessively about what others think of them.

Differential diagnosis: When is obsessive-compulsive disorder present?

- Medical history and developmental course: Developmental history is an important factor in differentiating OCD from ASD. OCD often presents in early childhood, typically before the age of three, and includes a wide range of symptoms, including social communication problems and restricted, repetitive behaviour patterns. OCD usually appears later, often in late childhood or early adolescence, and is characterised by specific, often newly occurring obsessive thoughts and actions.
- Diagnostic interviews and observations: The diagnosis of ASD is usually made using

comprehensive diagnostic interviews and standardised observation tools such as the Autism Diagnostic Observation Schedule (ADOS) or the Autism Diagnostic Interview-Revised (ADI-R). These instruments help to confirm the presence of ASD-specific symptoms such as deficits in social communication and restrictive, repetitive behaviour patterns. OCD, on the other hand, is typically diagnosed through clinical interviews and specific scales such as the Y-BOCS, which assess the presence and severity of obsessive thoughts and actions.

Reaction to treatment

The response to treatment approaches can also indicate the correct diagnosis. People with OCD usually respond well to cognitive behavioural therapy (CBT), particularly exposure therapy with response prevention (ERP). People with ASD often benefit from structured educational programmes, social support and behavioural therapy tailored to their specific developmental needs. If a person with rigid, repetitive behaviours does not respond to CBT, this could be an indication that ASD is present.

Overall, it is important that the diagnosis between OCD and ASD is made carefully, as both disorders require different treatment approaches. Accurate differentiation is crucial to ensure that sufferers receive the support they need to manage their specific symptoms and challenges.

5.3 Obsessive-compulsive disorder vs. depression

Obsessive-compulsive disorder and depression are two frequently comorbid disorders, but they are different in nature and symptoms. The distinction between these two disorders is crucial, as they require different therapeutic approaches.

Affective symptoms in comparison:

- Mood swings: Depression is characterised by a persistently depressed mood, anhedonia (loss of interest or pleasure in almost all activities) and a general feeling of hopelessness. People with depression often feel sad, worthless and lacking in energy. In OCD, depressive symptoms are often a reaction to the inability to control obsessive thoughts and the stress associated with them. While people with OCD may also experience depressive episodes, these are often secondary to the obsessive-compulsive symptoms.
- Thought content: In depression, thoughts are often characterised by self-deprecation, pessimism and feelings of guilt. People with depression often think about how worthless they are or how

bad the future is. In OCD, thoughts often centre around specific fears or anxieties that seem irrational, such as fear of contamination or constantly checking to see if a door is locked. These thoughts are intrusive and cause considerable anxiety, whereas depressive thoughts are characterised more by hopelessness and dejection.

Interactions and comorbidities:

- Comorbid depression in obsessive-compulsive disorder: It is not uncommon for people with OCD to also develop depressive symptoms, especially if the obsessive-compulsive symptoms are severe and severely interfere with daily life. The constant stress of obsessive thoughts and actions can lead to deep emotional exhaustion, which can lead to depression. This type of depression is often referred to as "reactive depression" as it occurs in response to the chronic stress of OCD.
- Influencing therapy: When depression and OCD occur at the same time, this can complicate treatment. For example, the listlessness and hopelessness that accompanies depression can make it difficult to focus on the cognitive behavioural therapy used to treat OCD. On the other hand, obsessive thoughts can exacerbate the course of depression by increasing feelings of overwhelm and hopelessness.

Diagnostic challenges and solutions:

- Differentiation of the main symptoms: Differentiating between the main symptoms of depression and OCD is crucial for an accurate diagnosis. While OCD focuses on specific obsessive thoughts and actions designed to relieve anxiety or discomfort, depression is characterised more by pervasive negative mood and anhedonia. It is important to recognise these differences in order to develop the right treatment strategy.
- Use of diagnostic tools: Validated questionnaires and clinical interviews are useful to help differentiate between depression and OCD. The Beck Depression Inventory (BDI) can be used to measure the severity of depressive symptoms, while the Yale-Brown Obsessive Compulsive Scale (Y-BOCS) helps to assess the severity of obsessive-compulsive symptoms. Combined use of these instruments may allow for a more accurate diagnosis.
- Therapeutic approaches: If both disorders occur simultaneously, a combination therapy may be necessary. Antidepressants such as SSRIs (selective serotonin reuptake inhibitors) are often used for both depression and OCD and can provide relief for both disorders. However, cognitive behavioural therapy (CBT) should be specifically targeted at the obsessive-compulsive symptoms

and depressive mood in order to treat both disorders effectively.

Overall, it is important that depression and OCD are carefully diagnosed and treated, as they are often linked and can influence each other. A comprehensive treatment strategy that takes both disorders into account is crucial in order to achieve effective symptom relief and improve the quality of life of those affected.

5.4 Obsessive-compulsive disorder vs. bipolar disorder

Obsessive-compulsive disorder and bipolar disorder are two mental illnesses that are sometimes difficult to distinguish from each other, especially when obsessive thoughts and actions occur in phases associated with bipolar disorder. Differentiating between these two disorders is crucial as they require different treatment methods.

Manic and depressive phases: Differentiation from obsessive-compulsive symptoms:

- Manic phases: In bipolar disorder, manic or hypomanic phases alternate with depressive phases. In a manic phase, those affected may show an exaggerated sense of self-worth, a reduced need for sleep, increased activity and risky behaviour. This symptomatology differs

significantly from obsessive-compulsive disorder, in which there are no episodes of euphoria or excessive energy. In manic phases, however, sufferers may exhibit compulsive behaviour motivated by impulsivity and increased risk-taking behaviour rather than anxiety or the need for control.
- Depressive phases: During the depressive phases of bipolar disorder, symptoms may resemble those of unipolar depression, including deep sadness, anhedonia and listlessness. Obsessive-compulsive disorder can be characterised by a worsening of obsessive thoughts and actions during these phases as emotional distress increases. The difference, however, is that OCD symptoms are specifically focused on the defence against anxiety and worry, whereas depression is characterised more by general hopelessness and despair.

Comorbid manifestations:

- Coexistence of obsessive-compulsive disorder and bipolar disorder: In some cases, obsessive-compulsive disorder and bipolar disorder can occur at the same time. This is known as a comorbid condition and requires special attention as the two disorders can influence each other. For example, obsessive-compulsive symptoms may increase during a manic phase as sufferers try to

control their excessive energy and impulsivity through ritualised actions. Similarly, the depressive phases of bipolar disorder can exacerbate obsessive thoughts and actions as the feeling of hopelessness increases.
- Differentiation of symptoms: In comorbid cases, it is important to clearly differentiate the symptoms of the two disorders. The manic and depressive episodes of bipolar disorder should be diagnosed using the classic criteria such as mood swings, activity levels and sleep patterns. Obsessive-compulsive symptoms should be assessed separately to determine whether they are indicative of an independent OCD or whether they occur in the context of the bipolar episodes.

Diagnostic differentiation and therapeutic approaches:

- Diagnostic criteria: The diagnosis of bipolar disorder is based on the identification of at least one manic or hypomanic episode alternating with depressive episodes. Obsessive-compulsive disorder, on the other hand, is diagnosed by the presence of recurrent obsessive thoughts and actions that cause significant anxiety and severely interfere with daily life. It is important that clinicians consider the possibility of a comorbid disorder and diagnose both disorders separately.
- Treatment: Treatment of bipolar disorder usually requires the use of mood stabilisers such as

lithium or anticonvulsants as well as antipsychotics to control manic episodes. When OCD is comorbid, SSRIs can be used to alleviate the obsessive-compulsive symptoms. Combination therapy, which includes both pharmacological and psychotherapeutic approaches, is often necessary to effectively treat both disorders. Cognitive behavioural therapy (CBT) can be particularly useful in reducing obsessive-compulsive symptoms, while psychotherapeutic interventions aimed at regulating mood are used to treat bipolar disorder.

Overall, the differentiation and treatment of OCD and bipolar disorder requires careful clinical assessment to ensure that both disorders are properly diagnosed and treated. Comprehensive, integrative therapy is often the key to success in improving the quality of life of those affected and preventing relapses.

5.5 Obsessive-compulsive disorders vs. anxiety disorders

Obsessive-compulsive disorder and anxiety disorders are closely related mental disorders that often have similar symptoms. Both are characterised by intense anxiety, but the nature of the anxiety and the associated behaviours differ, which makes it necessary to differentiate between them.

Fear as a common denominator?

- The role of anxiety in obsessive-compulsive disorder: In OCD, anxiety is often specific to the content of obsessive thoughts. These thoughts may include irrational fears of contamination, hurting others or forgetting an important task. Anxiety is directly linked to the obsessive thoughts and subsequent compulsive actions aimed at preventing the feared scenario or alleviating the anxiety.
- Anxiety disorders and diffuse anxiety: Anxiety disorders, such as generalised anxiety disorder (GAD) or panic disorder, are characterised by broad-based, often undirected anxiety. In GAD, for example, sufferers experience chronic, excessive worry about a variety of everyday events that is not triggered by specific obsessive thoughts. The anxiety is diffuse and can extend to numerous aspects of life without being alleviated by specific actions or rituals.

Specific differences in the symptoms:

- Ritualised actions vs. avoidance behaviour: A key difference between OCD and anxiety disorders lies in the type of behaviours used to cope with the anxiety. Obsessive-compulsive disorders focus on ritualised, compulsive actions that are intended to restore a sense of control and

security. In anxiety disorders, on the other hand, sufferers tend to avoid anxiety-inducing situations without performing specific rituals. For example, someone with social anxiety disorder might avoid social interactions, while someone with OCD might perform ritualised actions such as repeated hand washing to alleviate anxiety.
- Intrusiveness of thoughts: In obsessive-compulsive disorders, obsessive thoughts are typically intrusive and intrusive; they force their way into the sufferer's consciousness unintentionally and cause considerable discomfort. These thoughts are often alien and contradict the person's own beliefs. In anxiety disorders, on the other hand, the worries and thoughts are less intrusive and often appear as more realistic fears that exist in the context of everyday life.

Diagnostic criteria and differentiation:

- DSM-5 and ICD-10 criteria: The diagnostic criteria for OCD and anxiety disorders are clearly defined in the DSM-5 and ICD-10 and differ in terms of the type and focus of anxiety and the accompanying behaviours. Obsessive-compulsive disorder is diagnosed by the presence of obsessive thoughts and actions that cause significant anxiety and interfere with daily functioning. Anxiety disorders, on the other hand, are diagnosed by persistent, excessive fear and worry

that is not associated with specific obsessive thoughts.
- Clinical interviews and tests: Clinical interviews and specific questionnaires, such as the Generalised Anxiety Disorder 7 (GAD-7) for generalised anxiety disorder and the Yale-Brown Obsessive Compulsive Scale (Y-BOCS) for obsessive-compulsive disorder, can help to differentiate between the disorders. These instruments record the type of anxiety and the associated behaviours and can help to make an accurate diagnosis.
- Course and response to therapy: Another distinguishing feature is the response to therapeutic interventions. While cognitive behavioural therapy (CBT) can be effective for both disorders, treatment for OCD often focuses on exposure and response prevention (ERP) to reduce compulsive behaviours. For anxiety disorders, the focus is often on coping with worry through cognitive restructuring and improving coping strategies.

Differentiating between OCD and anxiety disorders is crucial for choosing the right therapeutic approach. While both disorders cause intense anxiety, they differ in the type of anxiety, the accompanying behaviours and the treatment. An accurate diagnosis is crucial in order to offer sufferers the best possible support.

5.6 Obsessive-compulsive disorders vs. sleep disorders

Sleep disorders can be both a symptom and a consequence of OCD, which makes the distinction between primary sleep disorders and sleep-related symptoms in OCD a diagnostic challenge.

Connection between sleep and obsessive-compulsive symptoms:

- Sleep disorders as a result of obsessive-compulsive disorder: People with OCD often report difficulty falling asleep or sleeping through the night due to the constant presence of obsessive thoughts. Sufferers can lie awake for hours worrying or performing obsessive behaviours that they cannot stop. These sleep disturbances can exacerbate the symptoms of OCD, as lack of sleep impairs the brain's ability to regulate emotions and make rational decisions.
- Impact of sleep on OCD symptoms: Lack of sleep can exacerbate OCD symptoms by increasing overall anxiety levels and impairing cognitive abilities. People who do not get enough sleep tend to be less able to control intrusive thoughts, leading to an increase in compulsive behaviours. Lack of sleep can also increase the risk of obsessive thoughts occurring, as the brain is more

susceptible to intrusive thoughts when in a depleted state.

Sleep problems as a consequence or symptom?

- Primary sleep disorders: Sleep disorders such as insomnia, sleep apnoea or restless legs syndrome (RLS) can occur independently of obsessive-compulsive disorder. These disorders have specific symptoms and causes that are not directly related to obsessive thoughts or actions. For example, insomnia is often caused by stress, depression or poor sleep hygiene, while sleep apnoea is caused by breathing problems during sleep. However, these primary sleep disorders can also exacerbate obsessive-compulsive symptoms if they disrupt sleep and increase overall anxiety levels.
- Sleep disorders caused by obsessive-compulsive symptoms: Sleep disorders in people with OCD are often a direct result of obsessive thoughts and actions. These sleep problems are usually secondary to the OCD symptoms and improve when the OCD is treated. For example, someone who spends hours obsessing before bedtime may have difficulty getting enough sleep, leading to daytime sleepiness and worsening of the obsessive-compulsive symptoms.

Differential diagnosis and treatment approaches:

- Diagnostic criteria: The distinction between primary sleep disorders and sleep-related symptoms in OCD requires a careful history and diagnosis. Primary sleep disorders usually have specific diagnostic criteria described in the DSM-5 and ICD-10. Obsessive-compulsive sleep disorders should be considered as secondary sleep problems caused by the underlying OCD.
- Polysomnography and sleep studies: If a primary sleep disorder is suspected, a polysomnography (sleep study) can be performed to analyse sleep patterns and diagnose disorders such as sleep apnoea or restless legs syndrome. These studies can help identify primary sleep disorders that may need to be treated before the obsessive-compulsive symptoms can be alleviated.
- Combined treatment approaches: If sleep disorders occur secondary to OCD, treatment should be aimed at reducing the symptoms of OCD. Cognitive behavioural therapy (CBT) can help to reduce obsessive thoughts and actions and thus improve sleep. For primary sleep disorders, specific interventions such as sleep hygiene training, medication or the treatment of sleep apnoea may be necessary.

Overall, it is important to consider sleep disorders and obsessive-compulsive symptoms as potentially related problems that require a combined diagnostic and therapeutic approach. Accurate diagnosis and tailored treatment can help to improve both sleep quality and obsessive-compulsive symptoms, leading to a better overall quality of life.

6. therapy and treatment of obsessive-compulsive disorders

6.1 Psychotherapy: approaches and techniques

Psychotherapy is a key form of treatment for OCD and has been shown to be highly effective, particularly in the form of cognitive behavioural therapy (CBT). This section explores the different psychotherapeutic approaches used to treat OCD and details the techniques used within these approaches.

Cognitive behavioural therapy (CBT):

- Exposure with response prevention (ERP): This is the most commonly used technique within CBT for the treatment of OCD. In exposure with response prevention, sufferers are deliberately confronted with the triggers of their obsessive thoughts without being allowed to perform their usual compulsive actions. For example, someone suffering from a cleaning compulsion could be asked to touch a contaminated surface and then refrain from washing their hands. The aim of this technique is to help sufferers learn that the feared consequences will not materialise even if they do not perform their compulsive actions. This leads to a gradual desensitisation to the

triggers and a reduction in obsessive-compulsive symptoms.
- Cognitive restructuring: This technique aims to identify the underlying beliefs and thought patterns that maintain the obsessive-compulsive symptoms. In cognitive restructuring, the therapist and patient work together to identify irrational and distorted thoughts and replace them with more realistic and functional thoughts. For example, a patient who believes that they can cause harm through their thoughts may learn to view these thoughts as unimportant and irrelevant, which reduces the intensity of the obsessive-compulsive symptoms.
- Mindfulness-based CBT: Mindfulness-based approaches combine traditional CBT techniques with mindfulness exercises. Mindfulness helps sufferers to notice and accept their thoughts and feelings without judgement, which can reduce emotional reactivity to obsessive thoughts. These approaches encourage sufferers to recognise their obsessive thoughts as "just thoughts" and not have to react to them, which leads to a reduction in compulsive behaviour.

Psychoeducation:

- Understanding the disorder: Psychoeducation is an essential part of the treatment of OCD. It involves educating sufferers about the nature of

their disorder, including its causes, symptoms and how treatment works. The aim is to help sufferers develop a better understanding of their disorder, enabling them to better control and manage their symptoms.
- Involvement of family members: Family members are often included in psychoeducation to help them understand their loved one's disorder and learn how to act in a supportive manner. Family members play an important role in the treatment process, especially when they learn how to avoid reinforcing the person's compulsive behaviour.

Depth psychology-based therapy:

- Focus on unconscious conflicts: While cognitive behavioural therapy is the gold standard in the treatment of OCD, depth psychology-based therapy offers a different approach. This approach focuses on exploring unconscious conflicts and past experiences that may have contributed to the development of OCD symptoms. The therapy aims to bring these unconscious conflicts to consciousness and process them in order to change the psychological mechanisms that maintain the obsessive-compulsive symptoms.
- Work on self-perception: Depth psychology-based therapy also emphasises the importance of self-perception and the development of a more

stable sense of self-worth. Many people with OCD have deep-rooted doubts about their own worthiness or their ability to have control over their lives. By working on these issues, therapy can help to reduce the need for compulsive behaviour.

Acceptance and Commitment Therapy (ACT):

- Acceptance of thoughts and feelings: Acceptance and Commitment Therapy (ACT) is another modern approach that focuses on accepting thoughts and feelings rather than trying to control or change them. In ACT, sufferers learn to accept their obsessive thoughts and feelings without attaching too much importance to them or reacting to them compulsively. This can lead to a reduction in obsessive-compulsive symptoms, as sufferers no longer feel the need to control their thoughts.
- Value-based actions: Another important aspect of ACT is the focus on values-based actions. The therapy encourages those affected to focus on what is really important to them in life and to take actions that are in line with these values, rather than spending their energy on controlling obsessive thoughts and actions.

Psychotherapy offers a variety of approaches and techniques that can be effective in the treatment of OCD. It is important that therapy is tailored to the individual needs of the sufferer in order to achieve the best possible results. Combining exposure with response prevention, cognitive restructuring and other therapeutic techniques can help to regain control over OCD symptoms and improve quality of life.

6.2 Drug treatment options

Medication plays an important role in the treatment of OCD, especially in combination with psychotherapy. They can help to reduce the intensity of obsessive-compulsive symptoms and make therapy more effective. In this section, the various medication options for the treatment of obsessive-compulsive disorder are described in detail.

Selective serotonin reuptake inhibitors (SSRIs):

- Mode of action: SSRIs are the most commonly prescribed class of antidepressants for the treatment of OCD. They work by blocking the reuptake of serotonin in the brain, thereby increasing the availability of this neurotransmitter. Serotonin plays an important role in regulating mood, anxiety and obsessive thoughts. By increasing serotonin levels, SSRIs can help to reduce the intensity of obsessive-compulsive symptoms.

- Common SSRIs: Commonly prescribed SSRIs include fluoxetine, sertraline, paroxetine, citalopram and escitalopram. These medications have been shown to be effective in the treatment of OCD and are often used as first-line treatment.
- Dosage and efficacy: A higher dosage is often required for the treatment of obsessive-compulsive disorder than for the treatment of depression. The dosage is gradually increased until a therapeutic effect is achieved. It can take several weeks for the full effect of SSRIs to be felt. Around 40-60% of patients respond to treatment with SSRIs, and a significant reduction in obsessive-compulsive symptoms can be achieved.
- Side effects: Like all medications, SSRIs can have side effects. Common side effects include nausea, insomnia, headaches, sexual dysfunction and weight gain. Usually these side effects are mild and temporary, but in some cases they can be persistent and require medication adjustments.

Tricyclic antidepressants (TCAs):

- Clomipramine: Clomipramine is a tricyclic antidepressant that has also been shown to be effective in the treatment of obsessive-compulsive disorder. It works in a similar way to SSRIs by inhibiting the reuptake of serotonin, but also has an effect on noradrenaline. Clomipramine was the first drug to be approved specifically for the

treatment of OCD and remains an option, especially when SSRIs are not effective.
- Side effects of TCAs: Tricyclic antidepressants have a wider range of side effects compared to SSRIs. These include dry mouth, constipation, blurred vision, weight gain and in some cases cardiovascular effects such as tachycardia. Because of these side effects, clomipramine is often only used when SSRIs have not been sufficiently effective.

Antipsychotics:

- Augmentation therapy: In cases where SSRIs alone are not sufficiently effective, low-dose antipsychotics can be added as augmentation therapy. Antipsychotics act on the dopaminergic system and can help to enhance the effect of SSRIs, especially in patients who do not respond fully to treatment.
- Common antipsychotics: Commonly used antipsychotics for augmentation in OCD include risperidone, aripiprazole and quetiapine. These medications have been shown to be effective in reducing OCD symptoms when taken in conjunction with SSRIs.
- Side effects of antipsychotics: Antipsychotics can cause a range of side effects including weight gain, sedation, extrapyramidal symptoms (e.g. tremors, rigidity) and metabolic changes such as

increased risk of diabetes. The decision to use antipsychotics should be carefully considered and patients should be closely monitored.

Benzodiazepines:

- Short-term use: Benzodiazepines such as diazepam, lorazepam or clonazepam are sometimes used for short-term relief of acute anxiety associated with obsessive-compulsive disorder. These drugs work quickly by increasing the activity of the neurotransmitter GABA, which has a calming effect. However, benzodiazepines are not suitable for the long-term treatment of OCD as they have a high potential for dependence and tolerance development.
- Side effects of benzodiazepines: In addition to the risk of dependence, benzodiazepines can also lead to drowsiness, concentration problems and coordination disorders. Their use should therefore be limited to acute crisis situations and under medical supervision.

Individual adjustment of medication:

- Personalised treatment approaches: Not all patients respond to the same medication and it may be necessary to try different types of medication to find the most effective treatment. Genetic

predisposition, medical history and possible side effects all play a role in the choice of medication.
- Combination therapies: In many cases, a combination of medications may be required to effectively treat the obsessive-compulsive symptoms. This may involve combining SSRIs with an antipsychotic or a TCA. Close collaboration with a specialist is crucial to find the optimal medication combination and dosage.

Long-term perspective:

- Duration of drug treatment: OCD is often a chronic disorder and medication may be necessary in the long term. Patients who respond well to medication may take it for several years to prevent relapses. Sudden discontinuation of medication can lead to a recurrence of symptoms, so medication should always be discontinued gradually and under medical supervision.
- Monitoring and adjustment: Drug therapy should be regularly reviewed and adjusted based on efficacy and side effects. It is important that patients are involved in the decision-making process and are informed about the advantages and disadvantages of the various treatment options.

Overall, medication is a central component of treatment for OCD. In combination with psychotherapy, it can help to alleviate symptoms and help sufferers to lead a normal life. Customised medication that is carefully monitored is the key to successful treatment.

6.3 Multimodal approaches: Combinations of forms of therapy

Multimodal approaches to the treatment of OCD combine various forms of therapy to ensure comprehensive and personalised treatment. This approach takes into account the complexity of the disorder and aims to treat both the psychological and physical aspects of the disorder.

Combination of psychotherapy and drug treatment:

- Synergy effects: The combination of psychotherapy, in particular cognitive behavioural therapy (CBT), with medication (e.g. SSRIs) has proven to be particularly effective in the treatment of OCD. While medication helps to reduce the intensity of obsessive thoughts and actions, CBT enables sufferers to develop strategies to deal with their symptoms and manage them in the long term.
- Indication-dependent combination: The decision as to which therapies should be combined depends on the severity of the OCD, the response to individual therapies and the patient's preference. In more severe cases, the combination of

SSRIs and CBT may be necessary, while in milder cases CBT alone may be sufficient.
- Extended psychotherapeutic approaches: In addition to CBT, other therapeutic approaches such as Acceptance and Commitment Therapy (ACT) or depth psychology-based therapy can be integrated into the multimodal approach. These approaches offer alternative perspectives and techniques that can be used depending on the specific needs of the patient.

Integration of alternative and complementary methods:

- Mindfulness and meditation: Mindfulness-based approaches such as mindfulness-based stress reduction (MBSR) and mindfulness-based cognitive therapy (MBCT) can be used as complementary therapies. These methods help those affected to develop a non-judgemental attitude towards their obsessive thoughts and feelings, which can lead to a reduction in obsessive-compulsive symptoms.
- Biofeedback and neurofeedback: Biofeedback and neurofeedback are technology-based approaches that help sufferers to monitor and control their physiological responses. These methods can be particularly helpful in the treatment of stress and anxiety associated with OCD. Neurofeedback, which aims to regulate brainwave

activity, can also be helpful in reducing obsessive thoughts and actions.
- Diet and exercise: The role of diet and exercise in the treatment of OCD is increasingly recognised. A balanced diet rich in nutrients such as omega-3 fatty acids, magnesium and vitamin D can stabilise mood and support the effectiveness of medication. Regular exercise, especially aerobic activities such as running or swimming, has been shown to have positive effects on mental health and can reduce the symptoms of OCD.

Coordination of multidisciplinary teams:

- Collaboration between professionals: A multimodal approach requires the close collaboration of a multidisciplinary team that includes psychotherapists, psychiatrists, primary care physicians, dietitians and other health professionals. These professionals must coordinate their efforts to ensure that the treatment plan is tailored to the patient's individual needs.
- Regular review and adjustment: The treatment of OCD is often a dynamic process that requires regular review and adjustment. Multimodal approaches make it possible to flexibly adapt the therapy based on the patient's progress, the occurrence of side effects or new findings about the effectiveness of certain interventions.

Long-term coping strategies:

- Prevention of relapse: Multimodal approaches also emphasise the importance of relapse prevention. This includes not only the continuation of medication and psychotherapy, but also training the patient in the use of coping strategies in everyday life. Mindfulness exercises, regular exercise and a balanced diet are crucial elements in preventing relapses.
- Promoting self-care: A key component of multimodal approaches is the promotion of self-care. Patients are encouraged to take an active role in their recovery by attending support groups, educating themselves about their disorder and taking proactive steps to promote their mental health.

Multimodal approaches offer a comprehensive, integrated treatment for OCD that is tailored to the individual needs of the patient. By combining different therapies and working together as a multidisciplinary team, more effective and sustainable treatment can be achieved.

6.4 Self-help and alternative treatment methods

Self-help and alternative treatment methods can be a valuable addition to conventional therapy for OCD. These approaches offer sufferers additional tools and strategies to manage their symptoms and improve their quality of life.

Self-help groups:

- Community support: Self-help groups offer sufferers the opportunity to share experiences with other people going through similar experiences. Sharing in a supportive community can reduce feelings of isolation and provide hope. In support groups, members share their experiences, discuss coping strategies and offer each other emotional support.
- Resources and information: Support groups are also often a source of useful information and resources, such as recommendations for therapists, books and articles about OCD, or techniques for coping with symptoms. These groups can help sufferers become better informed about their disorder and actively participate in their recovery.

Mindfulness and meditation:

- Stress management: Mindfulness and meditation practices can be an effective way to manage stress and reduce obsessive-compulsive symptoms. Mindfulness helps sufferers to observe and accept their thoughts and feelings without judgement, which can lead to a reduction in emotional reactivity to obsessive thoughts. Regular

meditation practice can help to reduce overall anxiety levels and improve the ability to cope with obsessive thoughts.
- Mindfulness-based stress reduction (MBSR): The MBSR programme, which consists of mindfulness-based physical exercises, meditation and mindfulness training, has been shown to be effective in reducing stress and improving mental health. Many people with OCD find MBSR techniques helpful tools to better manage their symptoms.

Nutrition and dietary supplements:

- Dietary changes: There is evidence that certain dietary habits can influence mental health. A diet rich in omega-3 fatty acids (e.g. from fish oil), magnesium, zinc and vitamin D can have positive effects on mood and brain function. A balanced diet can help to improve general well-being and support the effects of psychotherapy and medication.
- Dietary supplements: Some studies have shown that certain dietary supplements, such as N-acetylcysteine (NAC) or inositol, may be potentially useful in reducing obsessive-compulsive symptoms. NAC, an antioxidant that affects glutamate regulation in the brain, has shown promising results in some clinical trials. However, it is important to take such supplements only after

consulting a doctor, as they may interact with other medications.

Physical exercise:

- Mental and physical benefits: Regular physical exercise is not only good for your physical health, but also for your mental health. Exercise helps to reduce stress, release endorphins and improve overall mood. Activities such as running, swimming or yoga can lower overall anxiety levels and help reduce obsessive-compulsive symptoms.
- Yoga and bodywork: Yoga, which combines movement with breathing techniques and meditation, has been shown to be particularly useful in reducing anxiety and stress. Yoga promotes mindfulness, body awareness and relaxation, which are all factors that can help to alleviate obsessive-compulsive symptoms.

Creative therapies:

- Art and music therapy: Creative therapies such as art and music therapy offer alternative ways of expressing and processing emotions. These therapies can help to reduce inner tension and promote constructive ways of dealing with obsessive thoughts. Participating in creative activities can also boost self-esteem and provide a

positive distraction from obsessive-compulsive symptoms.
- Writing therapy: Writing can be a therapeutic activity that enables sufferers to organise and express their thoughts and feelings. Keeping a diary in which obsessive thoughts and actions are reflected upon can help to recognise patterns and develop strategies for coping.

Alternative healing methods:

- Acupuncture and acupressure: These traditional Chinese healing methods are sometimes used to relieve anxiety and stress. There is some evidence that acupuncture can restore balance in the body and help reduce OCD symptoms, although more research is needed to confirm its effectiveness for OCD.
- Homeopathy and herbal remedies: Some people turn to homeopathy or herbal remedies such as St John's Wort to relieve their symptoms. While these methods are found to be helpful by some, it is important to use them with caution and consult a doctor as herbal remedies can interact with other medications.

Long-term use and relapse prevention:

- Ongoing self-care: Self-help and alternative treatment methods should be seen as part of a

comprehensive, long-term plan for the treatment of OCD. These methods require commitment and regularity to be fully effective. Sufferers should feel encouraged to integrate these practices into their daily lives in order to achieve lasting improvement.
- Preparation for relapses: Although alternative treatments can be helpful, sufferers should prepare for possible relapses. Support groups and mindfulness training can be important tools for recognising and preventing relapses by taking early action if symptoms reappear.

Self-help and alternative treatment methods offer additional support for people with OCD and can help to complement conventional therapeutic approaches. These methods promote self-efficacy, strengthen well-being and offer sufferers additional tools to manage their symptoms.

6.5 Forecast and long-term management

The prognosis of OCD varies considerably from person to person and depends on several factors, including the severity of symptoms, early intervention and the quality of treatment. Long-term coping strategies are crucial to control symptoms and improve quality of life.

Long-term forecast:

- Chronic course: Obsessive-compulsive disorders are often chronic illnesses that can persist for many years without treatment. Symptoms can fluctuate over time, with phases of improvement and worsening. In severe cases, obsessive-compulsive disorder can be very restrictive and have a major impact on daily life.
- Positive treatment results: For many patients who receive appropriate treatment, particularly a combination of psychotherapy and medication, symptoms can be significantly reduced. With continued treatment and support, many people with OCD can learn to successfully manage their symptoms and lead a fulfilling life.
- Influence of comorbidities: Prognosis can be influenced by the presence of comorbid disorders such as depression, anxiety disorders or substance abuse. These additional disorders can complicate treatment and worsen the long-term prognosis, but require an integrated treatment strategy.

Relapse prevention:

- Long-term medication: In patients who respond well to drug treatment, it may be necessary to maintain the medication over a longer period of time in order to prevent relapses. Stopping the

medication abruptly can lead to a recurrence of symptoms, which is why the medication should be phased out gradually and under medical supervision.
- Continuation of therapy: Even after symptoms have improved, it is often advisable to continue therapy in order to prevent relapses. This can take the form of regular therapy sessions, refresher sessions or participation in self-help groups. Therapy can also help to develop new coping strategies when new challenges arise.
- Self-observation and early warning signs: Those affected should learn to recognise early warning signs of a relapse, such as an increase in obsessive thoughts or the need to resume old compulsive behaviours. By regularly observing themselves and defining a plan of action in the event of a relapse, those affected can take early action to prevent their symptoms from worsening.

Strategies for long-term coping:

- Lifestyle changes: A healthy lifestyle, including regular physical activity, a balanced diet and adequate sleep, can help manage OCD. These factors contribute to overall physical and mental health and can help reduce overall anxiety levels.
- Stress management: As stress is a major factor that can trigger or exacerbate obsessive-compulsive symptoms, learning stress management

techniques is crucial. Mindfulness exercises, meditation and relaxation techniques can help to reduce stress and strengthen emotional resilience.
- Social support: Building and maintaining a strong social network is an important part of coping with OCD in the long term. Family members, friends and support groups can provide emotional support that reduces feelings of isolation and strengthens motivation to continue treatment.

Maintaining the quality of life:

- Vocational and social rehabilitation: In severe cases where OCD has had a significant impact on life, vocational and social rehabilitation may be necessary. Programmes aimed at reintegrating sufferers into the labour market or helping them to re-establish social relationships can be invaluable.
- Self-acceptance and lifestyle: Long-term coping often requires lifestyle adjustments and acceptance that OCD can remain a part of life. This means having realistic expectations of yourself and focussing on what you can control. Accepting your own limits and setting achievable goals can help to boost self-esteem and lead a fulfilling life despite the disorder.

- Importance of a meaningful life: Dealing with questions of meaning and values can help to find a positive way of life despite the challenges of OCD. Activities that are perceived as meaningful, such as volunteer work, hobbies or setting personal goals, can strengthen the feeling of self-efficacy and enrich life.

Long-term management of OCD requires a holistic, sustainable approach that is tailored to the individual needs and circumstances of the person affected. With ongoing support, appropriate therapeutic approaches and active involvement in their own recovery, many people with OCD can lead fulfilling and productive lives.

7. prevention and education

7.1 Early detection and intervention

Early detection and intervention are crucial to positively influence the course of OCD and prevent symptoms from worsening. This section highlights the importance of early detection and the strategies that can be used for early intervention.

Importance of early detection:

- Prevention of chronicity: Early recognition of OCD can help to prevent the symptoms from becoming chronic. If OCD is diagnosed and treated early, there is a greater chance of effectively controlling the symptoms and maintaining the sufferer's quality of life.
- Reduction of comorbidities: Obsessive-compulsive disorders often occur together with other mental disorders such as depression, anxiety disorders or substance abuse. Early detection makes it possible to identify and treat these comorbid disorders at an early stage, which improves the overall prognosis.
- Relief for sufferers and families: Early intervention can reduce the level of suffering for both sufferers and their families. A quick diagnosis and the start of suitable treatment can help to reduce

the burden of the symptoms and help those affected to stabilise more quickly.

Strategies for early intervention:

- Screening programmes: The implementation of screening programmes in schools, universities and primary health services can help to identify OCD at an early stage. Such programmes could include standardised questionnaires such as the Obsessive Compulsive Inventory-Revised (OCI-R) or the Yale-Brown Obsessive Compulsive Scale (Y-BOCS) to help identify at-risk individuals.
- Educating the general population: Educating the general population about the symptoms of OCD is crucial to encourage early recognition. Campaigns in the media, information events and materials in healthcare facilities can raise awareness of OCD and increase the willingness to seek help.
- Training of professionals: Health and education staff should be trained to recognise early signs of OCD and respond appropriately. This includes training in the use of screening tools, raising awareness of symptoms and providing knowledge of appropriate referral pathways.

Obstacles to early detection:

- Stigmatisation: A significant obstacle to the early detection of OCD is the stigmatisation that is often associated with mental disorders. Sufferers and their families may be reluctant to seek help for fear of discrimination or social rejection. This can lead to symptoms being hidden or downplayed, making early detection difficult.
- Misinterpretation of symptoms: Obsessive-compulsive symptoms are often misunderstood or dismissed as "weird quirks", especially if they are mild. Both sufferers and relatives may have difficulty recognising the symptoms as signs of a serious mental disorder, which delays diagnosis.

Measures to promote early detection:

- Improving access to diagnostic services: Access to mental health services needs to be improved to ensure that people who may suffer from OCD can be diagnosed early and without barriers. This could include the establishment of dedicated counselling services, online diagnostic tools and the promotion of telehealth care.
- Promote self-help strategies: Self-help strategies and tools should be promoted to help sufferers recognise their symptoms and take early action. Validated self-tests, information leaflets and online resources can be important first steps to

raise awareness and encourage seeking professional help.

Early detection and intervention are key elements in minimising the long-term effects of OCD and improving the quality of life of those affected. By taking targeted measures to promote early detection, treatment can begin earlier and thus be more effective.

7.2 Prevention programmes and educational work

Prevention programmes and educational work are crucial to raising awareness of OCD, minimising risk factors and changing social perceptions. In this section, the various aspects of prevention and education are explained in detail.

Objectives of the prevention programmes:

- Reduction of risk factors: Prevention programmes aim to identify and minimise risk factors that could contribute to the development of OCD. These include genetic predispositions, environmental factors such as stress or trauma and psychological factors such as perfectionism or an excessive sense of responsibility.
- Promoting resilience: Another aim of prevention is to promote resilience, i.e. the ability to successfully cope with stress and challenges. Resilience

can be strengthened by teaching coping strategies, stress management techniques and promoting a healthy lifestyle.
- Early intervention for at-risk groups: Prevention programmes are also aimed at people who are at an increased risk of developing OCD, such as children of parents with OCD or people suffering from severe chronic stress. Targeted early intervention programmes can reduce the risk of developing OCD.

Types of prevention programmes:

- School-based prevention programmes: Schools are an ideal place to run prevention programmes as they have access to large numbers of young people. Programmes that focus on promoting mental health, reducing bullying and dealing with stress can help to reduce the risk of developing OCD. Lessons that address mental health can help to reduce stigmatisation and promote understanding of OCD.
- Workplace-related prevention programmes: Stress management and mental health programmes can be implemented in the workplace. These programmes can include stress management training, mindfulness training and workshops to promote a balanced lifestyle. Employers should be encouraged to create a supportive environment where employees feel comfortable

talking about their mental health and seeking support.
- Community-based prevention programmes: At the community level, prevention programmes can be run by local health organisations, support groups and community-based initiatives. These programmes can include talks, workshops and information sessions that raise awareness of OCD and provide support.

Educational work:

- Media campaigns: Media campaigns play an important role in educating the general public about OCD. Through the use of television, radio, print media and social media, information about the symptoms, causes and treatment options of OCD can be disseminated. Campaigns can also highlight stories of sufferers to promote understanding and empathy for people with OCD.
- Educational materials: The production and dissemination of educational materials such as brochures, flyers and online resources can help to increase knowledge about OCD. These materials should be easily accessible and understandable and aimed at sufferers, their relatives and the general public.
- Events and workshops: Events such as conferences, workshops and seminars provide opportunities to educate and share knowledge about

OCD. These events can bring together professionals, sufferers and their families to share information and discuss the latest research and treatment options.

Challenges in prevention work:

- Stigmatisation and prejudice: One of the biggest challenges in prevention and awareness-raising work is overcoming stigmatisation and prejudice against mental disorders. Many people still have misconceptions about OCD and are reluctant to seek help for fear of social rejection. Awareness programmes need to focus on combating these prejudices and creating a more open and understanding climate.
- Access to resources: In many regions, access to mental health services is limited, making it difficult to implement effective prevention programmes. It is important that prevention work is also accessible in rural and underserved areas to ensure that all population groups are reached.

Success criteria for prevention programmes:

- Evidence-based approaches: Prevention programmes should be based on evidence-based approaches that have been proven effective in research. Regular evaluation and adaptation of

programmes is necessary to ensure that they achieve the desired results.
- Inclusion and diversity: Prevention and education work should be inclusive and take into account the needs of different population groups, including different age groups, cultural backgrounds and social classes. Programmes should be sensitive to cultural differences and strive to reach all people.

Prevention programmes and educational work are crucial for raising awareness of OCD, minimising risk factors and changing social perceptions. Through targeted and evidence-based measures, these programmes can help to prevent the development of OCD and support those affected at an early stage.

7.3 Stigmatisation and social perception

OCD, like many other mental disorders, is often associated with a significant degree of stigmatisation. This stigmatisation can make life considerably more difficult for sufferers by creating barriers to seeking help, affecting self-esteem and leading to social isolation. This section examines the nature of stigmatisation of OCD and proposes measures to combat this stigma.

Nature and causes of stigmatisation:

- Misconceptions and myths: Many people have misconceptions about OCD, often caused by ignorance or misinformation. For example, the disorder is often misunderstood as a simple "exaggeration" of normal behaviours, such as excessive cleanliness or obsessive control. Such misconceptions can lead to OCD being seen as less serious or as something that sufferers could "just switch off" if they wanted to.
- Media portrayal: The way OCD is portrayed in the media can contribute to stigmatisation. People with OCD are often portrayed as "crazy" or "ridiculous" in films, TV programmes or news reports, which reinforces stereotypes and makes it more difficult to understand the complexity of the disorder.
- Social norms: Societal norms and expectations, particularly with regard to perfectionism and control, can increase the stigmatisation of OCD. In cultures that place a high value on order, cleanliness and discipline, OCD can be seen as extreme or inappropriate, which reduces the willingness of sufferers to talk about their symptoms or seek help.

Effects of stigmatisation:

- Barriers to help: Fear of stigmatisation can prevent sufferers from seeking professional help. Many people with OCD fear being seen as "crazy" by others if they disclose their symptoms, which leads them to hide their problems and not seek treatment.
- Social isolation: Stigmatisation can lead to social isolation, as sufferers may avoid talking about their disorder or socialising for fear of rejection or misunderstanding. This isolation can exacerbate symptoms and further impair quality of life.
- Worsening of symptoms: Stigmatisation can also lead sufferers to stigmatise themselves, which undermines their self-esteem and confidence in their own ability to deal with the disorder. This negative self-perception can intensify the obsessive-compulsive symptoms and reduce the willingness to participate in therapeutic measures.

Measures to reduce stigmatisation:

- Awareness campaigns: Awareness campaigns aimed at the general public are an effective way to reduce stigmatisation. These campaigns should focus on debunking myths about OCD, explaining the complexity of the disorder and sharing stories of sufferers to promote empathy and understanding.

- Training for professionals: Healthcare, education and social care professionals should be trained in recognising and dealing with OCD. Such training can help to reduce prejudice and ensure that sufferers receive the help they need in a supportive and non-judgemental environment.
- Involvement of those affected: Sufferers themselves should be encouraged to take part in awareness and anti-stigma initiatives. By sharing their experiences, they can help to raise public awareness and encourage other sufferers not to hide their symptoms.
- Changing media portrayal: It is important that OCD is portrayed realistically and sensitively in the media. Producers and scriptwriters should be encouraged to create more accurate and respectful portrayals of mental disorders that promote understanding and reduce stigmatisation.

Success criteria for anti-stigma measures:

- Measurable changes: Antistigma interventions should be regularly evaluated to measure their effectiveness. This can be done by conducting surveys on attitudes towards OCD, measuring the frequency of help-seeking or analysing the cross-media representation of the disorder.
- Sustainability of the initiatives: Sustainability is crucial to the success of anti-stigma initiatives. Measures should be designed for the long term

and continuously developed to ensure continued progress in reducing stigmatisation.

Stigmatisation remains a major challenge for people with OCD. However, through targeted education, the promotion of respectful representation in the media and the active involvement of those affected, an environment can be created in which OCD is better understood and accepted.

7.4 Importance of social support

Social support plays a crucial role in coping with OCD and can significantly improve the quality of life of those affected. This section examines the different forms of social support and their influence on the course and treatment of OCD.

Forms of social support:

- Emotional support: Emotional support includes the provision of comfort, understanding and empathy from friends, family and communities. It is important for people with OCD to have people around them who do not judge their experiences, but listen to them and encourage them. Emotional support helps those affected to feel less isolated and strengthens their ability to deal with the challenges of the disorder.

- Practical support: Practical support can take the form of help with everyday tasks or accompaniment to therapy sessions. As OCD is often associated with ritualised actions that take up a lot of time, practical support can help sufferers to manage their daily commitments while continuing their treatment.
- Informative support: Informative support involves sharing knowledge about OCD and possible treatment options. This form of support can be provided by therapists, self-help groups or by friends and family sharing literature and resources. Well-informed support people can help sufferers make informed decisions about their treatment and become better informed about their disorder.

Influence of social support on treatment success:

- Encouraging adherence to treatment: Social support can help to ensure that those affected continue their treatment and adhere to the recommended therapeutic measures. Supportive relationships provide encouragement and motivation, which is particularly important when treatment becomes difficult or emotionally stressful.
- Reduction of stress and anxiety: Access to a stable social network can lower overall stress levels and help to reduce the anxiety associated with

OCD. This can have a positive impact on symptoms and improve the effectiveness of treatment.
- Increased self-esteem: Social support can strengthen the self-esteem and self-efficacy of people with OCD. When sufferers feel valued and understood by those around them, this strengthens their confidence in their ability to deal with their disorder and regain control over their lives.

Challenges in providing social support:

- Lack of understanding in the social environment: Not all friends or family members understand the complexity of OCD, which can lead to misunderstandings and frustration. It is possible that support persons may unintentionally encourage behaviour that reinforces the obsessive-compulsive symptoms or that they have difficulty responding appropriately to the needs of the person affected.
- Emotional strain on the supporter: Providing ongoing support to a person with OCD can be emotionally draining, especially if progress is slow or setbacks occur. Support persons can feel overwhelmed or helpless, which can lead to burnout or conflict in the relationship.
- Balance between support and autonomy: It is important to find a balance between providing support and promoting the autonomy of the person

concerned. Excessive support can make the person concerned feel dependent and reduce their ability to cope on their own.

Strategies for effective social support:

- Education and training: Relatives and friends should be informed about OCD and the needs of those affected. Training and information materials can help to avoid misunderstandings and improve the ability to provide effective support.
- Support groups for relatives: Support groups for relatives offer a platform to share experiences, find support and learn from the strategies of others. These groups can help to reduce the emotional burden and provide practical tips for dealing with the situation.
- Promote self-care among carers: Relatives and friends should be encouraged to look after their own emotional and mental health. Taking regular breaks, setting boundaries and seeking your own support are important strategies for avoiding burnout and providing effective support in the long term.

Social support is a key factor in coping with OCD. By providing emotional, practical and informational support, the social environment can make a significant contribution to improving quality of life and treatment success. However, it is important to recognise the challenges associated with support and develop strategies to manage these effectively.

8 Conclusion and outlook

8.1 Summary of the key findings

This thesis has dealt extensively with the recognition and understanding of OCD, a mental illness that is widespread but often misunderstood in the general population. One of the key findings of this thesis is that OCD is a significant psychological burden that can severely affect the daily lives of those affected. They are characterised by the presence of obsessive thoughts, which are experienced as intrusive and unpleasant, and compulsive actions, which serve as attempts to cope with anxiety.

In the course of the work, it became clear that a clear and precise diagnosis of OCD is crucial in order to enable adequate treatment. The differentiation of OCD from other mental disorders such as ADHD, autism spectrum disorder, depression, bipolar disorder, anxiety disorders, sleep disorders, sensory processing disorders and schizophrenia is of great importance. This differentiation is often difficult, as there are symptomatic overlaps that can favour an incorrect diagnosis.

Another important result of the work is the emphasis on self-diagnosis as a first step in identifying OCD. However, it was made clear that self-diagnosis should only be considered as a supportive tool. Validated self-tests and questionnaires, such as the Yale-Brown Obsessive Compulsive Scale (Y-BOCS), can help to make an initial assessment, but the final diagnosis should always be made by a specialist or therapist.

The work has also shown that OCD is often associated with significant cognitive and emotional side effects, including anxiety, shame and guilt. These concomitant symptoms can exacerbate the symptoms and further impair the quality of life of those affected. The impact of OCD on behaviour and coping with everyday life was also investigated, and it became clear that the disorder leads to considerable restrictions in many areas of life, be it in the social, professional or family environment.

8.2 Future research directions and open questions

While working on the topic, several areas were identified where further research is needed. One of the most urgent tasks for future research is the improvement of diagnostic tools to facilitate the differentiation of OCD from other mental disorders. Although there are already established tests and diagnostic criteria, there is a need to further develop these instruments, especially with regard to their application in different cultural and social contexts. It would be of great benefit if future studies could focus on the cultural validity and cross-cultural adaptation of these instruments.

Another important area of research concerns the causes and mechanisms of OCD. Although the neurobiological and genetic basis is increasingly the subject of scientific research, the interplay between these factors and environmental influences has not yet been fully clarified. In particular, the role of epigenetic mechanisms and their influence on the development and course of OCD should be investigated in more detail in future studies. This research could help to develop preventive measures and identify potential risk groups at an early stage.

Digitalisation and the use of artificial intelligence (AI) also offer promising approaches to improve the diagnosis and treatment of OCD. Future research could focus on how digital technologies can be used in clinical practice to support diagnosis and develop personalised treatment strategies. For example, AI-supported systems could help to monitor symptoms and assess treatment success in real time. These technologies could also contribute to the development of digital therapies, which would be particularly useful in regions with limited access to psychotherapy services.

Another field of research concerns comorbidities, i.e. the co-occurrence of OCD with other mental or somatic illnesses. It is known that OCD often co-occurs with depression, anxiety disorders or eating disorders, which can significantly complicate treatment. Future research should focus on how these comorbidities can be better understood and integrated into therapy. Here, integrative therapeutic approaches that address both the OCD and the comorbid conditions could offer a promising perspective.

Another important issue is the stigmatisation of people with OCD. Although mental illness is increasingly moving into the public discourse, the stigmatisation of OCD remains a significant problem that can reduce the willingness to seek help. There is an urgent need for further studies that investigate how stigmatisation is perceived in different social groups and which strategies can effectively contribute to reducing prejudice. It would be particularly important to develop awareness campaigns that specifically target OCD and help to reduce public misconceptions.

Finally, the long-term effects of OCD on the quality of life and well-being of those affected should also be researched more intensively. Long-term studies could provide information on which factors favour successful coping with the disorder and how relapses can be avoided. These findings could help to further improve therapeutic approaches and ensure sustainable mental health for those affected.

8.3 Concluding remarks

This study has dealt intensively with the topic of obsessive-compulsive disorder and attempted to provide a comprehensive overview of the various aspects of this complex disorder. It became clear that OCD not only represents a considerable burden for those affected, but is also a challenge for diagnosis and treatment. Differentiating obsessive-compulsive disorder from other mental disorders is of crucial importance in order to ensure adequate and effective treatment.

A key contribution of this paper is that it emphasises the importance of self-diagnosis for the early detection of OCD, while at the same time highlighting the limitations of this method. Self-diagnosis can be a valuable tool for recognising the first signs of a disorder, but should always be carried out in combination with a professional diagnosis by a specialist or therapist.

The work also shows that there are still many unanswered questions and areas of research that need to be addressed in order to further deepen our understanding of OCD and improve treatment options. In particular, the role of digital technologies, research into comorbidities and the reduction of stigmatisation are areas in which future studies can make an important contribution.

In conclusion, it can be said that the work not only provides theoretical insights, but also highlights practical implications for the treatment and management of OCD. It provides a sound basis for further scientific research and can serve as a resource for professionals, sufferers and their families. The knowledge gained from the work should help to raise awareness of OCD, improve diagnosis and ultimately improve the quality of life of those affected.

The reader is encouraged not only to consider the knowledge gained in a theoretical context, but to actively put it into practice, whether by supporting sufferers, promoting awareness initiatives or actively participating in research. OCD is a serious challenge, but with the right knowledge and tools, much can be done to positively impact the lives of those affected and help them lead fulfilling and healthy lives.

9. further literature

1 American Psychiatric Association. (2022). *Diagnostic and Statistical Manual of Mental Disorders (DSM-5-TR)*. 5th edition, revised version. American Psychiatric Publishing.

   - This standard work offers comprehensive criteria for the diagnosis of obsessive-compulsive disorder and other mental illnesses, which is essential for a differential diagnosis.

2 Stein, D. J., & Fineberg, N. A. (Eds.). (2019). *Obsessive-Compulsive and Related Disorders*. Oxford University Press.

   - This book offers in-depth insights into the various forms of obsessive-compulsive disorder and discusses differential diagnostic aspects. It also deals with related disorders that are important for self-diagnosis.

3 Penzel, F. (2000). *Obsessive-Compulsive Disorders: A Complete Guide to Getting Well and Staying Well*. Oxford University Press.

   - A practice-orientated book that offers strategies for dealing with OCD as well as information on self-diagnosis. Differential diagnoses are also discussed.

4 Storch, E. A., & McKay, D. (Eds.). (2014). *Handbook of Treating Variants and Complications in Anxiety Disorders*. Springer.

- This manual contains sections on OCD and its treatment, including differential diagnostic considerations. Particularly useful for clinical use and self-help.

5 Abramowitz, J. S., McKay, D., & Taylor, S. (2008). *Clinical Handbook of Obsessive-Compulsive Disorder and Related Problems*. The Guilford Press.

- A comprehensive work that provides detailed information on the clinical presentation of OCD, its differentiation from other disorders and self-diagnosis.

6 Salkovskis, P. M. (Ed.). (2019). *Cognitive-Behavioural Treatment of Obsessive-Compulsive Disorder*. Springer.

- This book focuses on cognitive behavioural therapies for OCD and contains valuable sections on self-diagnosis and differential diagnosis.

7 Veale, D., & Willson, R. (2005). *Overcoming Obsessive Compulsive Disorder: A Self-Help Guide Using Cognitive Behavioural Techniques*. Robinson.

- A self-help book based on cognitive behavioural techniques. It offers insights into self-diagnosis and explains how to differentiate OCD from other disorders.

8 Koran, L. M. (2015). *Obsessive-Compulsive Disorder in Clinical Practice. Taylor & Francis.

- This book is aimed at clinicians, but also offers valuable information for sufferers on self-diagnosis and differentiation of OCD.

9 Tolin, D. F. (2016). *Doing CBT: A Comprehensive Guide to Working with Behaviors, Thoughts, and Emotions*. The Guilford Press.

- A comprehensive CBT manual that also covers obsessive-compulsive disorder. Includes sections on self-diagnosis and differentiation from similar disorders.

10 Mataix-Cols, D., Pertusa, A., & Leckman, J. F. (2007). *Obsessive-Compulsive and Related Disorders: A Comprehensive Survey. Oxford University Press.

- A comprehensive overview of OCD and related disorders, including sections on differential diagnosis and self-diagnosis.

11 Clark, D. A., & Beck, A. T. (2010). *Cognitive Therapy of Anxiety Disorders: Science and Practice*. The Guilford Press.

- This book provides in-depth insights into the cognitive therapy of anxiety disorders, including obsessive-compulsive disorder. It includes specific sections on differentiating OCD from other anxiety disorders.

12 Rachman, S. (2003). *The Treatment of Obsessions. Oxford University Press.

- A classic in the treatment of obsessive-compulsive disorder with a focus on obsessions. The book also sheds light on the differentiation between obsessive-compulsive disorder and other mental illnesses.

13 Baxter, L. R., Schwartz, J. M., Bergman, K. S., et al. (1992). *Caudate Glucose Metabolic Rate Changes with Both Drug and Behaviour Therapy for Obsessive-Compulsive Disorder*. Archives of General Psychiatry, 49(9), 681-689.

- This article examines the biological basis of OCD and shows how it differs from other mental disorders, which is relevant for accurate self-diagnosis.

14 Foa, E. B., & Kozak, M. J. (1997). *Mastery of Obsessive-Compulsive Disorder: A Cognitive-Behavioural Approach, Therapist Guide*. Oxford University Press.

- This guide for therapists is also useful for lay people who want to learn more about cognitive behavioural therapy for OCD, including how to differentiate it from other disorders.

15 Meyer, V. (1966). *Modification of Expectations in Cases with Obsessional Rituals*. Behaviour Research and Therapy, 4(4), 273-280.

- A groundbreaking article that demonstrates how expectation change can be effective in the treatment of OCD. This article is useful for understanding how OCD can be differentiated from other mental disorders.

16 Van Ameringen, M., Patterson, B., & Simpson, W. (2014). *Pharmacological Treatment of Obsessive-Compulsive Disorder: A Critical Review*. Current Pharmaceutical Design, 20(23), 3785-3799.

   - A critical overview of the pharmacological treatment of OCD, which also helps to understand pharmacological differences between OCD and other disorders.

17 Hyman, B. M., & Pedrick, C. (2005). *The OCD Workbook: Your Guide to Breaking Free from Obsessive-Compulsive Disorder*. New Harbinger Publications.

   - A practice-orientated workbook for sufferers that offers numerous self-help strategies and also contains information on self-diagnosis and differentiation from other disorders.

18 Abramowitz, J. S. (2006). *Understanding and Treating Obsessive-Compulsive Disorder: A Cognitive Behavioural Approach*. Routledge.

   - Another fundamental work on the cognitive behavioural therapy of obsessive-compulsive disorders, which also deals with the differentiation of similar disorders.

19 Fontenelle, L. F., Mendlowicz, M. V., & Versiani, M. (2006). *The Descriptive Epidemiology of Obsessive-Compulsive Disorder*. Progress in Neuro-Psychopharmacology and Biological Psychiatry, 30(3), 327-337.

- An important article on the epidemiology of obsessive-compulsive disorder, which helps to differentiate it from other mental illnesses.

20 Skoog, G., & Skoog, I. (1999). *A 40-Year Follow-Up of Patients with Obsessive-Compulsive Disorder*. Archives of General Psychiatry, 56(2), 121-127.

- A long-term study that provides valuable insights into the course of obsessive-compulsive disorder and helps to differentiate it from other long-term mental disorders.

21 Brockman, R., & Kamper, D. (Eds.). (2015). *The Wiley Handbook of Obsessive Compulsive Disorders*. Wiley-Blackwell.

- This comprehensive handbook covers all aspects of OCD, including diagnosis, differential diagnosis and treatment.

22 Wegner, D. M. (1989). *White Bears and Other Unwanted Thoughts: Suppression, Obsession, and the Psychology of Mental Control*. Viking.

- This book explores the phenomenon of thought suppression and its role in OCD, which is useful for understanding self-diagnosis and differentiation.